Eponyms in Surgery and Anatomy of the Liver, Bile Ducts and Pancreas

T0178880

Dedication

To my children, Paul, Catherine, and Stephen

Eponyms in Surgery and Anatomy of the Liver, Bile Ducts and Pancreas

Mark D Stringer BSc MS FRCP FRCS FRCS Paed, FRCSEd
Professor of Anatomy
Department of Anatomy and Structural Biology
Otago School of Medical Sciences
University of Otago
Dunedin, New Zealand

and

Former Professor of Paediatric Surgery and
Consultant Paediatric Hepatobiliary/Transplant Surgeon
St James's University Hospital
Leeds, UK

With assistance from

Seyed Ali Mirjalili MD
Assistant Research Fellow
Department of Anatomy and Structural Biology
Otago School of Medical Sciences
University of Otago
Dunedin, New Zealand

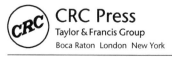

CRC Press
Taylor & Francis Group
Boca Raton London New York

CRC Press is an imprint of the
Taylor & Francis Group, an **informa** business

CRC Press
Taylor & Francis Group
6000 Broken Sound Parkway NW, Suite 300
Boca Raton, FL 33487-2742

First issued in paperback 2020

© 2009 by Taylor & Francis Group, LLC
CRC Press is an imprint of Taylor & Francis Group, an Informa business

No claim to original U.S. Government works

ISBN-13: 978-1-85315-985-5 (pbk)

Visit the Taylor & Francis Web site at
http://www.taylorandfrancis.com

and the CRC Press Web site at
http://www.crcpress.com

The right of Mark D Stringer to be identified as author of this work has been asserted by him in accordance with the Copyright, Designs and Patents Act, 1988.

British Library Cataloguing in Publication Data
A catalogue record for this book is available from the British Library.

Typeset by IMH(Cartrif), EH20 9DX, Scotland, UK

Contents

Contents

Foreword

This delightful book covers the eponyms used by those working in the field of HPB (hepatopancreatobiliary) surgery and the related anatomy. It includes all the famous names plus a few of those who may be less well known such as the anatomists Carl-Herman Hjortsjö from Lund in Sweden and Toshio Ito from Gumma in Japan. Hjortsjö's crook describes the angled course of the right posterior sectoral duct around an intrahepatic branch of the portal vein, while Ito's lipid-laden cells within the liver are also called hepatic stellate cells. The standard format adopted by Dr Stringer is to present the various eponymous conditions and then provide biographical details about the man whose name has been honoured, supplemented by key references and further reading. Diagrams, photographs and portraits embellish the text.

First in line for this treatment is John Abernethy. In my student days at St Bartholomew's Hospital, London I was President of the Abernethian Society, so I was ashamed to learn for the first time that he had described a variety of congenital extrahepatic portocaval shunt (the Abernethy malformation). Last to be described is Johann Wirsüng, who dissected out the pancreatic duct of an executed criminal in 1642 and engraved his findings on a copper plate. Alas the author did not survive to enjoy the fruits of his discovery that the pancreas was an exocrine gland, being slain in a private quarrel the following year. Copper plate and corpse remained in Padua, where dissection and murder were performed, although Wirsüng had been Bavarian by birth. Germany, France, the USA and Britain figure strongly among the countries that have nurtured HPB pioneers.

This book is a trove of fascinating information. Before reading it, I had thought that Calot's triangle was bounded by the cystic duct, the common hepatic duct and the lower border of the liver, and that it was crossed by the cystic artery. Not so: François Calot described the cystic artery, with or without the right hepatic artery, as the superior border of his triangle. Actually his real interest lay in orthopaedic surgery, and all four of his brothers were priests. Two of the subjects were ennobled, Berkeley Moynihan (cholecystectomy forceps) and Carl von Rokitansky (sinus, jointly with Karl Aschoff). Three were commemorated on postage stamps, Rokitansky for Austria, Kocher (incision, manoeuvre) for Switzerland and Laennec for France. Two were noted hunters, Arthur Mayo Robson (incision) who was accidentally shot in each thigh in Africa and Charles Puestow (operation) who is photographed as a U.S. army colonel in France after returning from la chasse in 1945.

As Wirsung's fate exemplifies, these eponym-bearers did not always have an easy life before being preserved for posterity. Thus Ruggero Oddi (sphincter) had to escape to the Congo following both a financial scandal and operations for appendicitis and intestinal obstruction. Later he returned to Belgium, only to become enmeshed in charges of quackery and die in Tunisia at the early age of 48 years. James Hogarth

Pringle (manoeuvre) lost all eight patients on whom he operated for blunt liver trauma, notwithstanding his attempts to occlude the vascular inflow. Ismar Boas (sign), who was of Jewish origin, was forced out of his post in Berlin by Hitler's racial oppression in 1936. He fled to Vienna, but killed himself after the German anschluss in 1938; to cap it all, his son was later killed by the Nazis; I now feel sorry that I have not looked more assiduously for cutaneous hypersensitivity below the right scapula in patients with acute cholecystitis.

George Grey Turner (sign) became first Director of Surgery at the Royal Postgraduate Medical School (RPMS) and the Hammersmith Hospital, London in 1935, and he held this post until 1945. Many years later I was destined to be the last Director of Surgery at these combined institutions before the RPMS was subsumed by Imperial College. I never met Grey Turner, who died in 1951, but I have met four of the other doctors highlighted in the book. One of the four is Henri Bismuth, while the other three I visited in the USA in 1979 as Moynihan Fellow of the Association of Surgeons of Great Britain and Ireland: Charles Frey (procedure), George Nardi (provocation test) and John Ranson (criteria of severity in acute pancreatitis). Later I wrote to Dr Nardi about a patient who developed acute pancreatitis after an injection of morphine and prostigmine and received a most courteous reply.

Reading the eponymous details provided in this book serves as an aide memoire to much of the history of HPB surgery, and Dr Stringer acts as an informative and entertaining guide. I have little doubt that others will find the book as enjoyable as I have done.

Professor Robin Williamson
MA MD MChir FRCS Hon DSc (Mahidol) Hon FRCS (Thailand)
President, Royal Society of Medicine, London, United Kingdom

Preface

For surgeons, physicians, and anatomists involved in the management and study of disorders of the liver, bile ducts and pancreas, eponyms are part of everyday communication. They help to describe anatomical features, operative procedures, surgical instruments, and diseases. Unfortunately, many have become distorted or are inaccurately applied. Few of us understand their derivation or the remarkable people and controversies behind them.

This book explores the origins of 70 eponyms in the field of hepatopancreatobiliary (HPB) surgery and anatomy. I began collecting material for this book almost five years ago, when I was a surgeon specialising in paediatric HPB surgery in the north of England and I continued to be interested in this field after moving into anatomy. Ali Mirjalili volunteered to become my research assistant in early 2008 and helped me complete the project, for which I am most grateful. I am indebted to the many surgeons and archivists from around the world who have generously provided material or checked biographical details during the last few years. I hope I have recorded them all in the Acknowledgements section of this book.

The focus of this monograph is on common eponyms in surgery and anatomy, rather than HPB disease. Each eponym is accompanied by a brief biographical sketch, which I hope gives a flavour of the person behind the eponym. I have deliberately avoided more comprehensive biographies, preferring instead to focus on the more interesting aspects of the person's life. References and further reading lists are supplied for those who would like to learn more. Where possible I have used primary sources and tried to corroborate important dates and facts. In so doing, I hope to minimise errors but readers should feel free to contact me if the record needs to be set straight.

The biliary tract is one of the most frequent sites of surgical intervention. In the United States alone, gallstone disease affects more than 20 million adults and cholecystectomy is among the top ten surgical procedures performed each year. In the United Kingdom, more than 50,000 such operations are performed annually. During the past 50 years, there has been a revolution in our understanding of hepatic anatomy and in the practice of liver surgery. Twenty years ago, few would have predicted that living-related liver transplantation would become a standard therapeutic option for end-stage liver disease. The pancreas has moved out of the obscurity of its retroperitoneal position and into the limelight, now that the benefits and limits of surgery on this organ are better understood.

I hope this monograph will enrich the reader's historical perspective of this fascinating branch of surgery and anatomy.

Mark Stringer

Acknowledgements

I am grateful to Sarah Ogden, Commissioning Editor at the RSM Press, who had the courage to support the publication of this book and who offered such helpful advice during production. I also wish to thank Robbie McPhee, Medical Illustrator and Graphic Artist in the Department of Anatomy and Structural Biology at the University of Otago, who expertly reformatted some of the images, and the staff of the Medical Library at the University of Otago, Dunedin for their efficient and friendly service.

There are numerous individuals and institutions deserving of special thanks for their help in providing material for this monograph.

Abernethy: Christine Woollett, Section Co-ordinator, Library and Information Services, The Royal Society, London, for permission to reproduce Abernethy's illustration of a congenital portocaval shunt (TabVII, p.66 from Abernethy J. Account of two instances of uncommon formation, in the viscera of the human body. Communicated by Sir Joseph Banks, Bart. P.R.S. Philosophical Transactions of the Royal Society of London 1793;**83**:59–66). Emma Butterfield, Picture Librarian, and Tom Morgan, Head of Rights and Reproductions at the National Portrait Gallery, London, for permission to reproduce the portrait of John Abernethy.

Bakeš: Dr Roman Šefr PhD, Associate Professor of Surgery, Masaryk Memorial Cancer Center, Brno, Czech Republic for the excellent background material on Jaroslav Bakeš.

Bismuth: Professor Henri Bismuth, Director of the Henri Bismuth Hepatobiliary Institute in Villejuif, France for supplying a portrait photograph.

Boas: Nancy Hulston, Director of the KUMC Archives, and Director of the Clendening History of Medicine Museum and Dawn McInnis, Rare Book Librarian, Clendening History of Medicine Library, University of Kansas Medical Center for their help with the portrait of Ismar Boas.

Budd: Rachael Cross, Picture Researcher, The Wellcome Trust, London for the lithograph of George Budd. Peter Coulson, General Secretary, Seamen's Hospital Society, Greenwich, London for the HMS Dreadnought engraving.

Burhenne: Dr Richard M Gore, President of the Society of Gastrointestinal Radiologists, Houston, Texas for permission to reproduce the photograph of Joachim Burhenne from the Society's website (http://www.sgr.org/).

Calot: Dr Christian Morin, Department of Pediatric Orthopedics, Calot Institute, Berck-sur-mer, France for his wonderful and varied pictures of François Calot and help in obtaining material from Calot's thesis. Thanks also to Dr Stephen J. Greenberg MSLS PhD, Coordinator of Public Services, History of Medicine Division, National Library of Medicine, National Institutes of Health, USA for the figure of Calot's triangle.

Carrel: Nicholas Scheetz, Manuscripts Librarian, Georgetown University Library Special Collections Research Center, Washington DC, USA for permission to reproduce the technique of vascular anastomosis from Carrel's original 1902 publication. Silka Quintero, Accounts and Permissions, The Granger Collection, New York for permission to use the photograph of Alexis Carrel operating during World War I.

Caroli: Gilles Colrat of Elsevier Masson SAS, Paris for permission to reproduce Figure 3, p.491 from Caroli J, Soupalt R, Kossakowski J, Plocker L, Paradowska M. La dilatation polykystique congenitale des voies biliaires intra-hepatiques. Essai de classification. *Semaine des Hôpitaux de Paris* 1958;**34**:488–95.

Charcot: Véronique Leroux-Hugon, Conservateur, Université Pierre et Marie Curie Paris VI, Service Commun de la Documentation Médicale, Bibliothèque Charcot, Hôpital de la Salpêtrière, Paris for kindly providing the image of Jean Martin Charcot.

Chiari: Zoe Harland, Assistant Librarian and Andrew Crymble, Reader Services Librarian, Royal Society of Medicine for providing access to Chiari H. Ueber die selbständige Phlebitis obliterans der Hauptstämme der Venae hepaticae als Todesursache. *Beiträge zur Pathologischen Anatomie und Zur Allgemeinen Pathologie* 1899;**26**:1–18, and the Royal Society of Medicine Library for allowing reproduction.

Couinaud: Thanks to Dr Francis Sutherland, Department of Surgery, University of Calgary, Canada for permission to reproduce the photograph of Claude Couinaud.

Courvoisier: Professor Holger Dathe of the Deutsches Entomologisches Institut, Müncheberg, Germany for kindly providing the portrait of Courvoisier; Dr Daniel Burckhardt of the Naturhistorisches Museum, Basel, Switzerland for donating the images from Courvoisier's butterfly collection; and Bianca Ruehling of Goettingen State and University Library, Germany for providing the title page of Courvoisier's monograph of 1890.

Child: Lucinda Cooke, Assistant Director Emeritus Faculty Services, University of Michigan Medical School for the portrait and obituary of Dr Charles G Child 3rd. Dr Nicholas Pugh, Consultant Public Health Physician, for his biographical details.

Cullen: The Alan Mason Chesney Medical Archives of The Johns Hopkins Medical Institutions for permission to reproduce the oil painting of Thomas Cullen.

Deaver: Dr James L Mullen MD, Chief of Surgery, University of Pennsylvania for the images of John Blair Deaver, and Donna Muldoon for permission to reproduce these. Daniel Peters, Leander, Texas for the image of the Deaver retractor.

Desjardins: Marie-Françoise Garreau, Université Pierre et Marie Curie, Service Commun de la Documentation Médicale, En mission au Musée Dupuytren-Fondation Dejerine, Paris for her expert assistance with background information. Thanks also to Jean-François Vincent, Conservateur, Chef du service d'histoire de la médecine, Bibliothèque Interuniversitaire de Médecine et d'odontologie, Paris for the image of Desjardins.

Disse: Kornelia Drost-Siemon, Ethik und Geschichte der Medizin Bibliothek, Georg-August-Universität Göttingen for her help with the photograph of Joseph Disse, and Karin Keller, Archivist at the University of Halle, Germany for permission to reproduce the image. Thanks also to Cornelia Pfordt, Librarian at Niedersächsische Staats-und Universitätsbibliothek, Schriftliche Auskunft/Historisches Gebäude, Göttingen, for the illustration from Disse's 1890 manuscript and permission to reproduce this.

DuVal: Matthew Wiencke, Assistant Editor, *Dartmouth Medicine* magazine, Lebanon, New Hampshire for kindly providing the photograph of Merlin DuVal.

Frey: Dr Charles F Frey MD FACS for his valuable insights into the development of the Frey procedure for chronic pancreatitis and permission to include his photograph.

Gans: Dr Henry Gans MD for generously sharing information about the fissure of Gans, for checking biographical details, and for kindly providing a photograph.

Glisson: Emma Shepley, Curator of the Heritage Centre, Royal College of Physicians, London for the portrait of Francis Glisson. Thanks also to the Brotherton Collection, Leeds University Library for access to Glisson's *Anatomia Hepatis*.

Grey Turner: Louise King, Assistant Archivist, The Royal College of Surgeons of England for the photographs of George Grey Turner. Christine Cowan, Walton Library, Faculty of Medical Sciences, Newcastle University for background information. Jessica Silver, Assistant Archivist and Records Manager, Corporate Records Unit and College Archives, Imperial College London for the photograph of Professor Grey Turner in the operating theatre circa 1936 (the photographer of this image is unknown but will be credited in any future reproduction should their identity become known).

Hartmann: Marie Davaine, conservateur en chef, Responsable des fonds anciens et iconographiques, Bibliothèque de l'Académie Nationale de Médecine, Paris for the portrait of Henri Hartmann. Thanks also to Professor Vincent Delmas, Président de la Société Anatomique de Paris for permission to reproduce the figure of Hartmann's pouch.

Hjortsjö: Gunnar Lundin, Medical Faculty Library, University of Lund for her generous assistance in obtaining images of Carl-Herman Hjortsjö and the Institute of Anatomy in Lund.

Ito: Dr Robert Kyle Pope, Chief of Electron Microscopy, Pathology Division, US Army Medical Research Institute of Infectious Diseases, Frederick, Maryland, USA for the photomicrograph of an Ito cell. Also to Allan Mitchell, Technical Manager, Otago Centre for Electron Microscopy, Department of Anatomy and Structural Biology, Otago School of Medical Sciences, University of Otago, Dunedin, New Zealand for help with this search.

Kasai: Professor Ryoji Ohi, Miyagi Children's Hospital, Sendai, Japan for the figures related to Morio Kasai.

Klatskin: Florence Gillich of the Cushing/Whitney Medical Historical Library, Yale University for help with the clinical photograph of Dr Klatskin. Stefanie Knab of Light, Inc. for her help in obtaining the photograph of Gerald Klatskin from the National Library of Medicine.

Kocher: Professor Urs Boschung, Institut fuer Medizingeschichte, Universitaet Bern, Switzerland for help with information on Theodor Kocher.

Kupffer: Sulo Lembinen, Manuscripts and Rare Books Department, University of Tartu Library, Tartu, Estonia for the photograph of Kupffer.

Langerhans: Norbert Ludwig, Picture Research, bpk Photo Agency, Fine Art, Culture and History, Berlin, Germany, for the photograph of Paul Langerhans.

LeVeen: Robert LeVeen MD, FACR, Associate Professor of Radiology, Shands Hospital, University of Florida for generously providing photographs of his father, Harry LeVeen and to Betsy Waters, Executive Director, MUSC Office of Alumni Affairs, Medical University of South Carolina, Charleston, South Carolina for kindly putting me in contact with Dr Robert LeVeen. Thanks also to Monica Sanders, Director of Global Marketing, Interventional Specialties, CardinalHealth, Illinois, USA for the photograph of the Denver shunt and associated permission to reproduce it.

Lilly: Professor R Peter Altman, Surgeon-in-Chief at the Morgan Stanley Children's Hospital at the New York Presbyterian Hospital, Columbia University Medical Center, New York for checking John Lilly's biographical details and providing a photograph. Also to Wendy Cowles Husser MA MPA, Executive Editor, *Journal of the American College of Surgeons*, for permission to use the illustration of Lilly's technique.

Longmire: The Longmire Surgical Society, David Geffen School of Medicine at UCLA for permission to reproduce the photograph of William Polk Longmire Jr. Thanks also to Dr William Traverso MD, FACS, Virginia Mason Medical Center, Seattle, Washington, USA, who kindly checked the factual content of Longmire's biographical sketch. Finally, thanks to Jennifer Jones, Rights Assistant, Global Rights Department at Elsevier Ltd. for her help with securing permissions.

Lund: Special thanks to Torben V Schroeder MD DMSc, Professor of Vascular Surgery, Rigshospitalet, Copenhagen, Denmark, for his identification of the source of this eponym. Thanks also to the Boston Public Library for biographical information and to Harvard University Archives, Pusey Library, Cambridge, Massachusetts for the images of Fred Bates Lund.

Luschka: Ulrike Mehringer of Universitätsbibliothek Tübingen for kindly providing the photograph of Luschka and the figure of the bile duct from his 1863 publication. Thanks also to Professor Jean de Ville de Goyet and Mr Khalid Sharif of Birmingham Children's Hospital, UK for kindly providing the cholangiographic images of Luschka's duct.

Mirizzi: Professor Jorge Cervantes MD FACS (Hon), Professor of Surgery, National University of Mexico, American British Cowdray Medical Center, for kindly providing the photograph of the oil painting, the portrait photograph and background material on Pablo Mirizzi. Thanks also to Andrew Morgan, Library Assistant, The Royal College of Surgeons of Edinburgh for his help with background literature.

Morison: Cheryl Bell, Medical Photography Department, Royal Victoria Infirmary, Newcastle upon Tyne, UK for the image of the bronze plaque. Thanks also to Christine Cowan, Walton Library, Faculty of Medical Sciences, Newcastle University, Newcastle upon Tyne for assistance with background information on Morison.

Moynihan: Jim Garretts, Senior Curator, Thackray Museum, Beckett Street, Leeds, UK for kindly providing the images of Moynihan's cholecystectomy forceps.

Murphy: Mary Kay Stallone of the Chicago Surgical Society Central Office for her assistance with background information and the portrait photograph of John B Murphy.

Nardi: Suzanne Williams, Executive Assistant to Andrew L Warshaw MD, Surgeon-in-Chief and Chairman, Department of Surgery, Massachusetts General Hospital, Boston for the photograph of George Nardi.

Ochsner: Jack Simpson, Reference Librarian, Local and Family History, The Newberry Library, Chicago, Illinois, USA for Edward Ochsner's obituary. Kevin O'Brien, UIC Library of the Health Sciences Special Collections Department, Chicago, for additional biographical information. Erin Tikovitsch, Rights and

Acknowledgements

Reproductions and Jay Crawford, Photographer, Chicago History Museum for the photograph of Edward Ochsner.

Oddi: Susanna Mattioli of the Biblioteca Centr. and Professor Adolfo Puxeddu, Preside della Facoltà di Medicina e Chirurgia, Università degli Studi di Perugia for kindly providing the article and figure of Oddi's sphincter. Thanks also to Stefanie Knab of Light, Inc. for her help in obtaining the photograph of Ruggero Oddi from the National Library of Medicine.

Puestow: Philip Skroska, Archivist, Visual and Graphic Archives, Bernard Becker Medical Library, Washington University School of Medicine for the military photograph of Charles Puestow.

Pringle: James Beaton, Librarian, The Royal College of Physicians and Surgeons of Glasgow, for the portrait of Pringle and Andrew Connell, Museum Collections Manager, Royal College of Surgeons of England for kindly providing background material.

Ranson: H. Leon Pachter MD FACS, The George David Stewart Professor and Chair, Department of Surgery, NYU School of Medicine for kindly providing the photograph of John Ranson.

Retzius: Barbara Klockare, Culture Council, Karolinska Institutet, Stockholm, Sweden for permission to reproduce the portrait of Anders Retzius. Thanks also to Gunnar Lundin, Medical Faculty Library, University of Lund, for finding background information.

Rex: Professor Oldřich Eliška of the Institute of Anatomy, First Faculty of Medicine, Charles University in Prague for the portrait photograph and background information on Hugo Rex. Thanks also to Dr Jens Stahlschmidt, Consultant in Paediatric Pathology, St James's University Hospital, Leeds for his generous help with translation.

Riedel: Helga Seidel and Hans-Juergen Hillesheim of Thüringer Universitäts- und Landesbibliothek, Friedrich Schiller University of Jena, Germany for kindly providing the photograph of Bernhard Riedel and associated biographical background information.

Rokitansky: Dr Jens Stahlschmidt, Consultant in Paediatric Pathology, St James's University Hospital, Leeds, UK for kindly providing the photomicrograph of a Rokitansky–Aschoff sinus.

Roux: Eloi Contesse, Département des collections photographiques, Musée historique de Lausanne for the photograph of César Roux.

Saint: Warda Brown, Administration Officer, Groote Schuur Hospital, Cape Town, South Africa for the photograph of Charles Saint.

Santorini: Hilary Lane, History of Medicine Library Coordinator, Mayo Foundation, Rochester, Minnesota for the illustrations from Santorini's *Anatomici Summi Septemdecim Tabulae* by Michael Girardi (1775). Also thanks to Nina Rivers for her translation of Cagnetto G. *Un grande anatomico della Serenissima (Giandomenico Santorini)*. Atti del Reale Instituto Vemto di Scienze 1915–16; Tomo LXXV:1163–1188. Carlo Ferrari: Venezia.

Sengstaken: Jennifer McGillan, Archivist, and Stephen E. Novak, Head, Archives and Special Collections, Augustus C. Long Health Sciences Library, Columbia University Medical Center, New York, USA for the biographical information and images of Robert Sengstaken and Arthur Blakemore.

Sugiura: Professor A Yamataka, Department of Pediatric General and Urogenital Surgery, Juntendo University School of Medicine, Tokyo, Japan for the helpful biographical information and photograph of Mitsuo Sugiura. Thanks also to Kayleigh Harris, Rights Assistant, Elsevier Ltd for her prompt assistance with permission to reproduce Figure 1 from Sugiura and Futagawa's cited publication.

Vater: Anna-Elisabeth Bruckhaus, Universitaetsbibliothek Tübingen, Germany for the title page of Vater's 1720 manuscript.

Warren: Kathy Torrente, Health Sciences Center Library, and Barry Glasser, Business Manager, Department of Surgery, Emory University School of Medicine, Atlanta, Georgia for the photograph of Dean Warren.

Whipple: Dr Samir Johna MD FACS, Department of Surgery, Loma Linda University School of Medicine, California, USA for the photograph of Whipple.

Wirsüng: Professor Renato G. Mazzolini, Dipartimento di Scienze Umane e Sociali, Università degli Studi di Trento, Trento, Italy for generously providing key background literature on Wirsüng; Lucia Nardo, Servizio Cerimoniale e Manifestazioni, Università degli Studi di Padova, Italy for the image of Wirsung's original copper plate engraving and the image by Giacomo dal Forno; Giulia Rigoni Savioli, Librarian, Biblioteca Pinali antica, University of Padua for her search for relevant images and for introducing me to other helpful contacts; and the Photo Archive of the Messenger of Saint Anthony, Padua, Italy for the photograph of Wirsüng's cenotaph.

Introduction

So mind your Qs and mind your Ps;
Say "Thank you, sir," and "If you please."
Then some day, in the future dim,
You too may be an eponym.

Attributed to Willard R Espy (1910–1999), US writer and poet

"Those who cannot remember the past are condemned to repeat it."

George Santayana (1863–1952), poet and philosopher

What is an eponym?

Originating in the mid-nineteenth century, the term eponym is derived from two Greek words: *epi*, meaning 'upon', and *onama*, meaning 'a name'. The original definition of eponym referred to the person after whom a discovery, object, place or phenomenon was named or thought to be named (Pearsall 1998) but the term is now more commonly used as a noun describing the object associated with the name giver.

Should eponyms be abolished?

Are surgical and anatomical eponyms more trouble than they are worth? Purists maintain that all eponyms in surgery and anatomy should be abolished, regarding them as inaccurate and confusing, with no intrinsic descriptive value (Organ and Sojka 1961; Woywodt and Matteson 2007). One reason for this view is that eponyms are prone to distortion and misrepresentation with repeated use over the years, rather like the game in which each player successively whispers to the next person what he or she believes was whispered to them. For example, in hepatopancreatobiliary (HPB) surgery and anatomy, Calot's triangle is often used to describe that region in the right upper quadrant of the abdomen bounded by the cystic duct, common hepatic duct and undersurface of the liver. Although this region is of immense practical significance during cholecystectomy, this was not what François Calot originally described.

Eponyms can wrongly credit discovery to a particular individual or encourage us to overlook the major contributions of others. For example, the main pancreatic duct may have been identified first by Hoffman rather than Wirsüng and the accessory pancreatic duct by Rhode rather than Santorini (Stern 1986). However, in these and many other cases, the individual associated with the eponym was nevertheless usually the first to give the structure or object the prominence it deserved.

Many other reasons have been put forward for rejecting eponyms. These include: more than one eponym being associated with the same object (sometimes varying between countries); the same name used to designate different entities (e.g. Cooper's ligament can refer to part of the inguinal ligament or the suspensory ligaments of the breast); the perpetuation of historical inaccuracies (Organ and Sojka 1961); the eponym may not indicate the first, or even the most significant person involved with the object (Jeffcoate 2006); and the fact that eponyms usually refer to one person, whereas scientific discoveries often represent the effort of many (Woywodt and Matteson 2007).

Some have even ventured to state that eponyms provide a less than truthful account of discovery, and are too heavily determined by influence, politics, language, or sheer luck (Woywodt and Matteson 2007). Whilst this may be true to some extent, isn't this the case for all discoveries?

A more powerful argument for abolishing eponyms is that rarely they can be confused with potentially serious consequences. Paul Langerhans (1847–1888) was the first to describe not only the islets in the pancreas but also the antigen-presenting dendritic cells (now called Langerhans cells) of the skin. Theodor Langhans (1839–1915) was the German pathologist who first described the multinucleate cells, now known as Langhans cells, characteristic of the granulomas of tuberculosis. Descriptions of both Langerhans' dendritic cells and Langhans' giant cells appeared in the same journal, *Virchow's Archives*, in the same year (1868). In 2003, Pritchard and colleagues reported two instances in which the close resemblance between the names of these two eponymous cells led to misdiagnosis and inappropriate treatment (Pritchard et al 2003). In one, this was because of a typographical error in a histopathology report, and in the other there was a misunderstanding by the responsible clinician. In both cases, these errors led to damaging treatment for the wrong disease — tuberculosis instead of Langerhans' cell histiocytosis and vice versa.

Why preserve eponyms?

Although there are many flaws with the use of eponyms, this is not so much the fault of the eponym but more the consequence of human error and misinterpretation. Eponyms are so widely used in the English language that their eradication would be virtually impossible. Consider the following examples used in everyday speech: silhouette (Etienne de Silhouette), boycott (Captain Boycott), nicotine (Jean Nicot), masochism (Leopold von Sacher-Masoch) (Ruffner 1977), sandwich (John Montagu, 4th Earl of Sandwich), cardigan (James Brudenell, 7th Earl of Cardigan), diesel (Rudolf Diesel), joule (James Joule), biro ballpoint pen (László Biro) and hertz (Heinrich Hertz).

Eponyms frequently provide a convenient shorthand way of expressing complex phenomena, a fact that partly explains their abundance in medicine and the natural

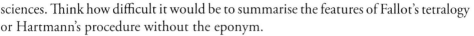

sciences. Think how difficult it would be to summarise the features of Fallot's tetralogy or Hartmann's procedure without the eponym.

Whether we like it or not eponyms are here to stay. Eponyms move in and out of the language of medicine with time and their shelf-life is determined by their usefulness. They are part of our surgical and anatomical heritage, adding both colour and humanity. They can also facilitate learning and recall. Their use acknowledges the contribution of those who helped to make anatomy and surgery what it is today.

In anatomy, eponyms are becoming less frequent with the emphasis on using the descriptive anatomical term as defined in *Terminologia Anatomica* (Federative Committee on Anatomical Terminology 1998). The latest edition of *Gray's Anatomy* (Standring 2008) still retains reference to many eponyms but it seems that it is only a matter of time before many disappear. In general surgery, many standard surgical instruments are designated by eponyms. With the reduction in training times in surgical training schemes, lack of knowledge of these is an increasing problem (Khwaja et al 2005). Some of the many eponyms in general surgery (Ellis 1983) will undoubtedly be lost but, hopefully, the useful ones will survive.

There have been a few occasions when major efforts to change the name of an eponym have been made. Thus, the American College of Chest Physicians believes that Wegener's granulomatosis should no longer be referred to by its eponym because of Friedrich Wegener's major involvement with the Nazi party before and during World War II (Lefrak and Matteson 2007; Woywodt and Matteson 2007). Exactly the same argument has been used to recommend that Hans Reiter (1881–1969) be dissociated from the condition of postinfective inflammatory mucositis and arthritis (Jeffcoate 2006). But, as Whitworth (2007) states: "...history is what happened, not what we or the revisionists wish had happened. We remember the names of tyrants and despise them, not celebrate them. Telling people what they must or must not say or write is fraught with danger."

An ongoing debate

The contrasting views about whether we should keep eponyms or not have been highlighted in recent years in two leading medical journals. Between 2000 and 2006, *The Lancet* ran a series of articles exploring selected eponymous medical conditions and the individuals behind these. The *British Medical Journal* debated the issue in 2007. Judging by the responses to that debate, most correspondents were in favour of retaining eponyms.

Eponyms in hepatobiliary and pancreatic surgery and anatomy

In HPB surgery and anatomy, eponyms have been attached to anatomical features, clinical signs, pathological disorders, diagnostic tests, surgical instruments, syndromes, operations, and manoeuvres. The vast majority of these seem to be both useful and

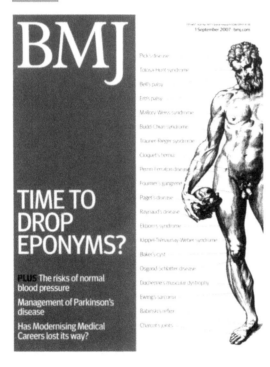

Front cover of the *British Medical Journal* 1 September 2007, Vol. 335. Reproduced with permission from the BMJ Publishing Group

appropriate. None include the individual's Christian name. Two of the surgeons were Nobel prize winners – Theodor Kocher (1909) and Alexis Carrel (1912) – quite an achievement considering that only nine surgeons have received this award since 1901 (Cosimi 2006; Toledo-Pereyra 2006).

The aim of this monograph is to bring together common eponyms in HPB surgery, in an attempt to give an accurate account of their origin. Not all eponyms are included – the focus is on surgery and anatomy rather than disease. For example, von Hippel–Lindau disease, Zollinger–Ellison syndrome, Frantz tumour and Wilson's disease are not included but Caroli's disease/syndrome and Laennec's cirrhosis are mentioned. Much as Tom Starzl (Starzl 1992) and Sir Roy Calne richly deserve to have some aspect of liver transplantation enshrined in an eponym, the plan when writing this book was to stick to common eponyms. A few selected instruments have been included but the list is far from comprehensive. Each eponym is accompanied by a brief biographical sketch, which gives a flavour of the person behind the eponym. For some individuals, biographical details have been difficult to obtain, especially since the eponyms span several centuries and many continents. Where possible I have used primary sources and tried to corroborate important dates and facts. In so doing, I hope to minimise errors but readers should feel free to contact me if the record needs to be set straight. I have deliberately avoided writing more comprehensive biographies, preferring instead to focus on the more interesting aspects of the person's life. However, I have included additional references for those who want to learn more. The use of the possessive in eponyms in general is variable, the North American trend being towards the non-possessive (Jana et al 2007). This monograph attempts to reflect common usage, e.g. Calot's triangle and Carrel patch.

The table tries to put a few of the eponymous discoveries featured in this monograph in the context of the history of medicine. Not surprisingly, the surgical

Selected eponyms in surgery and anatomy of the liver, bile ducts and pancreas in the context of the history of medicine

Year of publication	Discovery/publication	Originator/Country of origin
1543	De Humani Corporis Fabrica	Vesalius/Italy
1564	Use of ligatures to control bleeding	Paré/France
1628	Circulation of the blood	Harvey/England
1642	Pancreatic duct	Wirsüng/Italy
1654	Anatomia Hepatis	Glisson/England
1720	Hepatopancreatic ampulla	Vater/Germany
1775	Accessory pancreatic duct	Santorini/Italy
1803	Morphine isolated from crude opium	Sertürner/Germany
1809	First successful elective laparotomy (ovariotomy)	McDowell/USA
1829	First successful blood transfusion	Blundell/England
1832	First intravenous saline infusion	Latta/Scotland
1846	Ether anaesthesia	Morton/USA
1867	Antisepsis	Lister/UK
1869	Pancreatic islets	Langerhans/Germany
1881	First successful gastrectomy	Billroth/Austria
1882	First cholecystectomy	Langenbuch/Germany
1886	Ampullary sphincter	Oddi/Italy
1887	First successful planned liver resection	Langenbuch/Germany
1889	Successful choledochotomy	Abbe/USA and Knowsley Thornton/England)
1895	X-rays	Roentgen/Germany
1898	Pancreaticoduodenectomy	Codivilla/Italy
1901	ABO blood groups identified	Landsteiner/Austria
1902	Technique for vascular anastomosis	Carrel/France
1935	Sulphonamide antibiotics	Domagk/Germany
1957	Detailed liver segmental anatomy	Couinaud/France
1967	Successful liver transplant	Starzl/USA
1985	Laparoscopic cholecystectomy	Mühe/Germany
1989	Successful living-donor liver transplant	Strong/Australia

eponyms date more to the nineteenth and twentieth centuries whilst many of the anatomical discoveries were in the seventeenth and eighteenth centuries. In her excellent book on John Hunter, Wendy Moore (2005) provides a fascinating insight into the world of eighteenth century anatomy, commenting that "Across Europe, anatomists vied to discover and name previously unmapped parts of the body, staking their claim to a piece of the human interior. Intrepid anatomists could be assured of immortality through the parts they described; if they did not themselves bestow their names on their discoveries they could be certain their disciples would arrange that honour. .... so anatomists squabbled for priority in their discoveries. Often their claims and counter-claims could be exceedingly difficult to determine. The advent of printing and the development of high-quality plate engraving helped in allowing rival researchers to publish and display their findings, but in a period long before authoritative peer-reviewed scientific journals, and when anatomy books were beyond the pocket of many ordinary practitioners, anatomists also chose alternative ways of announcing their achievements."

These comments are borne out by many of the older eponyms included in this book.

References

Cosimi AB. Surgeons and the Nobel Prize. *Arch Surg* 2006;**141**:340–8.

Ellis H. *Bailey and Bishop's Notable Names in Medicine and Surgery.* 4th edition. HK Lewis, London, 1983.

Federative Committee on Anatomical Terminology. *Terminologia Anatomica: international anatomical terminology.* Thieme, Stuttgart, 1998.

Jana N, Barik S, Arora N. Eponyms deserve a uniform dressing, not a total shredding. *BMJ* 2007 http://www.bmj.com/cgi/eletters/335/7617/424#175614 (Last accessed December 2008).

Jeffcoate WJ. Should eponyms be actively detached from diseases? *Lancet* 2006;**367**:1296–7.

Khwaja N, Khwaja S, Murray D, Wong J, Murphy MO, Ghosh J. Trainees' knowledge of eponymous names for surgical instruments. *Ann R Coll Surg Engl* (Suppl) 2005;**87**:284–5.

Lefrak SS, Matteson EL. Friedrich Wegener. The past and present. *Chest* 2007;**132**:2065.

Moore W. *The Knife Man.* Bantam Press, London, 2005, pp96–7.

Organ CH, Sojka LA. The eponym problem. *Am J Surg* 1961;**102**:1–2.

Pearsall J. *The New Oxford Dictionary of English.* Clarendon Press, Oxford, 1998.

Pritchard J, Foley P, Wong H. Langerhans and Langhans: what's misleading in a name? *Lancet* 2003;**362**:922.

Ruffner JA. *EDI Eponyms Dictionaries Index.* Gale Research Co., Detroit, 1977.

Standring S. *Gray's Anatomy: the anatomical basis of clinical practice.* 40th edn. Elsevier, Philadelphia, 2008.

Starzl TE. *The Puzzle People: Memoirs of a Transplant Surgeon.* University of Pittsburgh Press, Pittsburgh, 1992.

Stern CD. A historical perspective on the discovery of the accessory duct of the pancreas, the ampulla 'of Vater' and *pancreas divisum. Gut* 1986;**27**:203–12.

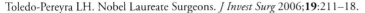

Toledo-Pereyra LH. Nobel Laureate Surgeons. *J Invest Surg* 2006;**19**:211–18.

Whitworth JA. Should eponyms be abandoned? No. *BMJ* 2007;**335**:425.

Woywodt A, Matteson E. Should eponyms be abandoned? Yes. *BMJ* 2007;**335**:424.

Further reading

Barsoum N, Kleeman C. Now and then, the history of parenteral fluid administration. *Am J Nephrol* 2002;**22**:284–9.

Blumgart LH. Resection of the liver. *J Am Coll Surg* 2005;**201**:492–3.

Ellis H. *A History of Surgery*. Greenwich Medical Media Ltd., London, 2001.

Glenn F, Grafe WR. Historical events in biliary tract surgery. *Arch Surg* 1966;**93**:848–52.

Howard JM, Hess W. *History of the Pancreas; mysteries of a hidden organ*. Kluwer Academic, New York, 2002.

McClusky III DA, Skandalakis LJ, Colborn GL, Skandalakis JE. Hepatic surgery and hepatic surgical anatomy: historical partners in progress. *World J Surg* 1997;**21**:330–42.

Abernethy malformation – congenital extrahepatic portocaval shunt

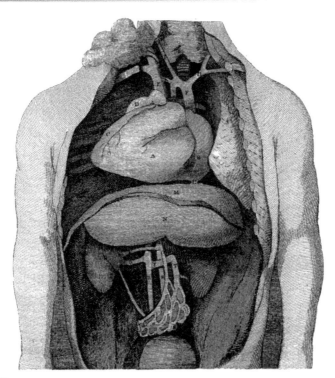

Abernethy malformation. L, hepatic vein; N, liver; O, superior mesenteric artery; P, renal artery; R, inferior vena cava; S, aorta; T, portal vein. (Reproduced by kind permission of The Royal Society, London. From Abernethy J. Account of two instances of uncommon formation, in the viscera of the human body. Communicated by Sir Joseph Banks, Bart. P.R.S. *Philos Trans R Soc Lond* 1793;**83**:59–66, TabVII, p.66)

In his 1793 article, Abernethy reported a 10-month-old female infant with the following congenital anomalies: dextrocardia; an interrupted inferior vena cava with azygos continuation; the confluence of hepatic veins draining directly into the right atrium; a portal vein that terminated in the inferior vena cava at about the level of the renal veins; an enlarged common hepatic artery (the sole blood supply of the liver); a central liver; an umbilical vein that drained into a hepatic vein; a small gall bladder containing bile (as did the transected bile duct); and polysplenia ('seven separate portions'). The cause of death in this infant was unknown but presumed due to an infectious disease.

The illustration from this article clearly shows a congenital extrahepatic end-to-side portocaval shunt. Several other varieties of congenital portosystemic venous shunts are now known to exist (Stringer 2008).

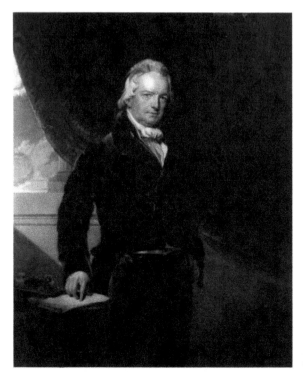

Portrait of John Abernethy FRS by the artist Sir Thomas Lawrence (1819–1820). (Reproduced with permission of the National Portrait Gallery, London)

John Abernethy (1764–1831)

John Abernethy was the son of a London merchant and grandson of a controversial minister in the Irish Presbyterian Church. At the age of 15 years, Abernethy was apprenticed to Sir Charles Blicke, Surgeon at St Bartholomew's Hospital in London, where he attended the surgical lectures of Percival Pott (1714–1788). He learnt anatomy and pathology from John Hunter (1728–1793), who influenced him greatly. In 1787, Abernethy was appointed Assistant Surgeon at St Bartholomew's Hospital but did not become Full Surgeon until 1815, and was never independently in charge of wards there. Despite this, he was widely respected by his peers, and was elected President of the Royal College of Surgeons of England in 1826 and became a Fellow of the Royal Society. He was instrumental in the founding of St Bartholomew's Medical School in 1822.

Abernethy was an accomplished and popular lecturer in anatomy, physiology and surgery. In 1791, St Bartholomew's Hospital built a lecture theatre especially to accommodate the pupils attracted by him. According to one pupil, "His lectures were full of original thought, of luminous and almost poetical illustrations, the tedious details of descriptive anatomy being occasionally relieved by appropriate and amusing anecdotes." At the time, doctors jealously guarded their hospital lectures in order to attract students and earn their fees. However, Thomas Wakley, founding Editor of *The Lancet* maintained that all lectures should be public property. The journal began sending reporters into the lecture halls and started publishing Abernethy's lectures verbatim in 1824, which led to a row between Abernethy and *The Lancet* and a temporary injunction on the journal. Subsequently, the matter was settled in favour of *The Lancet* in the courts.

By all accounts, Abernethy was a good surgeon, although understandably often reluctant to operate due to the high mortality rate of surgery at that time. Nevertheless, he was the first surgeon to tie the external iliac artery for popliteal aneurysm in 1797, extending John Hunter's pioneering work. He published on a wide range of topics in surgery, pathology and anatomy, including an article on the anatomy of the whale in 1796. He was renowned for his brusque manner with patients and his abhorrence of verbosity. When a patient came to his clinic holding up his index finger: "Burn?" asked Abernethy. "No, bite," said the patient. "Dog?" asked Abernethy; "Parrot," replied the patient. The consultation ended with a few simple directions for treatment.

Abernethy married the daughter of a widowed patient of his in 1800, after a less than romantic courtship. In his autobiography, Samuel Gross, a pioneering American surgeon, quoted Abernethy's proposal of marriage thus: "I have witnessed your devotion and kindness to your mother. I am in need of a wife, and I think you are the very person that would suit me. My time is essentially occupied, and I have therefore no leisure for courting... Reflect upon this matter until Monday." The woman subsequently became Mrs Abernethy and they had two daughters.

In 1828, the year before he retired, Abernethy became involved in a public scandal. He promised his support for an applicant to the staff of St Bartholomew's Hospital in return for cash and other favours, a practice that was apparently common among leading London surgeons at the time. This was exposed in *The Lancet*, reactivating old wounds. This episode is somewhat at odds with his character; although he received various honours, he was scornful of riches and rank and according to Thornton's biography, declined a baronetcy. He died in Enfield, North London at 67 years of age.

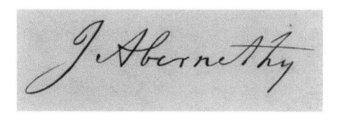

References

Stringer MD. The clinical anatomy of congenital portosystemic venous shunts. *Clin Anat* 2008;**21**:147–57.

Abernethy J. Account of two instances of uncommon formation in the viscera of the human body. Communicated by Sir Joseph Banks, Bart. P.R.S. *Philos Trans R Soc Lond* 1793;**83**:59–66.

Further reading

Gross SD. Autobiography of Samuel D Gross, MD with sketches of his contemporaries. Edited by his sons. George Barrie, Philadelphia, 1887.

Home E, Abernethy J. Some particulars in the anatomy of a whale. *Philos Trans R Soc Lond* 1796;**86**:27–33.

John Abernethy 1764–1831. *Br J Surg* 1913;**1**:549–50.

Macilwain G. *Memoirs of John Abernethy*. Hurst & Blackett, London, 1853.

Past Presidents. 3. John Abernethy. *Ann R Coll Surg Engl* 1950;**7**:505–7.

Thornton JL. John Abernethy and operative surgery. *J Bone Joint Surg (Br)* 1951;**33B**:636–41.

Thornton JL. *John Abernethy: A Biography*. Simpkin Marshall Ltd, London, 1953.

Williams DI. Portraits of a confrontation: Abernethy and Lawrence. *Ann R Coll Surg Engl* 1994(Suppl);**76**:14–17.

A Arantius duct or ligament

The ductus venosus connects the left branch of the portal vein in the fetus to the termination of the left hepatic vein, allowing oxygenated blood from the placenta to bypass the fetal liver and enter the inferior vena cava just below the right atrium. It is sometimes referred to as the Arantius duct or, since it typically closes soon after birth, the Arantius ligament.

The duct of Arantius is a useful landmark during liver splitting procedures in paediatric living donor liver transplantation (Majno et al 2002) and in extended left hepatectomy (Povoski et al 1999; Glick et al 2000).

According to Huisman and Wladimiroff (1993), the first and second editions of Arantius' book did not contain a description of the ductus venosus – this only appeared in the 1571 edition. These authors maintain that Andreas Vesalius first described this vessel in his last work *Anatomicarum Gabrielis Fallopii Observationum Examen*, published in 1564.

Giulio Cesare Aranzi (1530–1589)*

Also known as **Julius Caesar Arantius**, Giulio Cesare Aranzi was an Italian professor of surgery and anatomy at the University of Bologna. Based on his observations in human fetuses, he wrote *De Humano Foetu Libellus* in 1564. Aranzi is also credited with being the first to identify the levator palpebrae superioris muscle, coining the term 'hippocampus', and discovering the ductus arteriosus.

*No image of Arantius exists in the Historical Archives of the University of Bologna (Professor Gian Paolo Brizzi, Director).

References

Arantii GC. *De humano foetu libellus*. Bologna: Sacris Medicorum ac Philosophorum, Collegiis Bononiae. Ex officina Joannis Rubrii ad insigne Mercurii 1564.

Glick RD, Nadler EP, Blumgart LH, La Quaglia MP. Extended left hepatectomy (left hepatic trisegmentectomy) in childhood. *J Pediatr Surg* 2000;**35**:303–7.

Majno PE, Mentha G, Morel P, et al. Arantius' ligament approach to the left hepatic vein and to the common trunk. *J Am Coll Surg* 2002;**195**:737–9.

Povoski SP, Fong Y, Blumgart LH. Extended left hepatectomy. *World J Surg* 1999;**23**:1289–93.

Huisman TWA, Wladimiroff JW. The ductus venosus. *Fetal Mat Med Rev* 1993;**5**:45–55.

B Bakeš dilators

These malleable olive-type dilators come in a range of sizes and can be used to test the patency of the common bile duct and duodenal papilla and to determine the position of the latter during open operations on the bile duct. They can also be used as a guide when performing a sphincteroplasty.

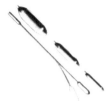

Bakeš dilators

In his 1923 publication on choledochoscopy, Bakeš described a series of dilators ranging from 1–14 mm in diameter for dilating the duodenal papilla. However, he probably first mentioned his dilators in 1902, when he was in Berlin (personal communication from Dr Roman Šefr).

Jaroslav Bakeš (1871–1930)

Jaroslav Bakeš was born near Brno in the Czech Republic. His father was a teacher and his mother the daughter of a local doctor.

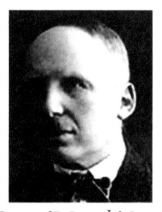

Jaroslav Bakeš. (Courtesy of Dr Roman Šefr, Brno, Czech Republic)

Bakeš studied medicine in Vienna, graduating in 1895. After postgraduate training in Vienna he returned to the Czech Republic and in 1909 was appointed Chief of Surgery at the regional hospital in Brno. Bakeš was a general surgeon, making notable contributions in the fields of colorectal surgery, neurosurgery, and biliary

7

tract surgery. He designed numerous surgical instruments and provided the earliest report of choledochoscopy using a rigid instrument. Much of his surgical wisdom was distilled into a textbook on surgical techniques and results, published in 1927.

Bakeš was a recognised surgical leader in the Czech Republic. He operated on the goitre of the mother of the world famous Czech compositor Leoš Janáček. In close cooperation with the first president of Czechoslovakia, Dr Tomáš Garrique Masaryk, he founded a 'House of Consolation' for the treatment of cancer patients in 1935. The Bakeš Memorial Surgical Hospital in Brno was founded in 1922 but closed in 2006, when it became part of Masaryk Memorial Cancer Center and is now called Bakeš Pavilion.

In addition to his work, Bakeš had a passion for hunting. He died from pneumonia during a hunting trip to Poland. Bakeš cousin, Karel Absolon (1877–1960), a famous archaeologist and cave researcher, celebrated Jaroslav Bakeš' achievements in a book devoted to a millennium of culture in Czechoslovakia.

References

Bakeš J. Die choledochopapilloskopie, nebst Bemerkungen über Hepaticusdrainage und Dilatation der Papille. *Arch Klin Chir* 1923;**126**:473–83.

Further reading

Absolon KB. Jaroslav Bakeš, Surgeon, Naturalist, and Philanthropist. In *Czechoslovakia Past and Present*, Volume 2. Mouton, The Hague, 1968, pp1632–42.

Olivero R, Penka I, Sefr R, Trávnícek F. The multi-talented surgeon, Dr Jaroslav Bakeš. *Rozhl Chir* 1996;**75**:553–6 (in Czech).

B Baumgarten recess

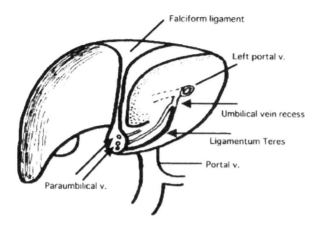

A diagrammatic illustration of the umbilical vein recess (Baumgarten recess). (From Hashimoto M, Heianna J, Tate E, et al. Small veins entering the liver. *Eur Radiol* 2002;**12**:2000–5, Fig. 1 © European Society of Radiology, Vienna. With permission of Springer Science & Business Media)

The umbilical vein is connected to the left branch of the portal vein in the fetus but is usually occluded in adults, forming the ligamentum teres. A variable length (up to 10 cm) of the terminal segment of this vein may remain patent in normal individuals. This is known as the Baumgarten or umbilical vein recess and may connect with paraumbilical vein(s) in the falciform ligament. It is usually small but can be prominent in patients with portal hypertension. Reference to the recess is mostly found in the ultrasound or angiographic literature on portal hypertension.

Paul Clemens von Baumgarten (1848–1928)

He was a German pathologist who worked at the anatomical institutes in Leipzig and Königsberg and later became Professor of Pathological Anatomy and General Pathology at the University of Tübingen. He is best known for his identification of the tubercle bacillus in 1882, which he discovered independently of Robert Koch, but his publication appeared a few weeks after Koch had announced his discovery in Berlin.

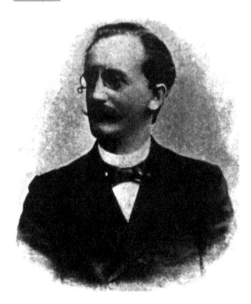

Paul Clemens von Baumgarten.

Baumgarten's name is also associated with Cruveilhier–Baumgarten disease/syndrome, which was described by the French anatomist Jean Cruveilhier (1791–1874) in 1852 and by von Baumgarten in 1907 (von Baumgarten 1907). This condition comprises prominent patent umbilical and paraumbilical veins associated with a venous hum and occurs in patients with portal hypertension and splenomegaly, with or without liver cirrhosis.

References

Hashimoto M, Heianna J, Tate E, et al. Small veins entering the liver. *Eur Radiol* 2002;**12**:2000–5.

von Baumgarten P. Ueber vollständiges offenbleiben der Vena umbilicalis; zugleich ein Beitrag zur Frage des Morbus BantPaul Clemi. *Arb Geb Pathol Anat Inst Tübingen* 1907;**6**:93–110.

Further reading

Bisseru B, Patel JS. Cruveilhier–Baumgarten (C–B) disease. *Gut* 1989;**30**:136–7.

Steinberg JS, Galambos JT. Cruveilhier–Baumgarten (C–B) disease. An experiment of nature. *Am J Med* 1967;**43**:284–8.

Yeh HC, Stancato-Pasik A, Ramos R, Rabinowitz JG. Paraumbilical venous collateral circulations: color Doppler ultrasound features. *J Clin Ultrasound* 1996;**24**:359–66.

Bismuth classification of postoperative bile duct strictures

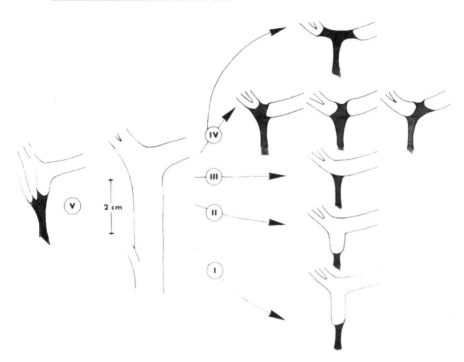

Types of postoperative bile duct strictures classified according to the length of the residual proximal bile duct. Three landmarks are used: 2 cm below the biliary confluence, the inferior level of the confluence, and the roof of the confluence.

Five types of bile duct strictures were recognised:

Type I: Low common hepatic duct stricture – residual hepatic duct longer than 2 cm

Type II: Middle common hepatic duct stricture – residual hepatic duct less than 2 cm

Type III: High stricture or hilar stricture preserving the biliary confluence. The stricture extends to the confluence of the right and left hepatic ducts but communication between the two hepatic ducts is preserved at this level.

Type IV: Hilar stricture interrupts the confluence – communication between left and right branches no longer exists.

Type V: A stricture involving an anomalous arrangement of the segmental right branches.

(Reprinted with permission from Bismuth H. Postoperative strictures of the bile duct. In Blumgart LH (ed). *The Biliary Tract*, Churchill Livingstone, Edinburgh, pp209–18 © 1982).

11

Bismuth's classification of postoperative bile duct strictures was first reported in 1981 in French literature and became well known after it was published in English the following year. Bismuth divided bile duct strictures according to the site of obstruction and the length of the residual proximal duct, both factors being major determinants of repair and outcome. In the original classification, based on a national study of 643 cases of postoperative biliary stricture, cholecystectomy had been the primary operation in 92% of cases. Three varieties of clinical presentation were described: progressive jaundice, an external biliary fistula, and biliary peritonitis with or without cholangitis. The long-term complication of secondary biliary cirrhosis was also highlighted. In the 1982 article, Bismuth went on to describe the principles of repair of these strictures: establishing bilio-enteric drainage with a healthy, wide, tension-free mucosa-to-mucosa anastomosis (Bismuth et al 1982). The use of the Hepp–Couinaud technique of lowering the hilar plate to improve exposure of the left hepatic duct for anastomosis was also emphasised.

Bismuth subsequently refined the classification slightly, incorporating isolated right hepatic duct strictures. After the introduction of laparoscopic cholecystectomy in the late 1980s, the Bismuth classification formed the basis for the description of iatrogenic bile duct injuries.

Henri Bismuth (1934–)

Henri Bismuth is Director of the Henri Bismuth Hepatobiliary Institute in Villejuif, France and a renowned hepatobiliary surgeon. He pioneered liver transplantation in Europe. Among his many accomplishments, he was the first to perform a liver transplant in France and the first to use reduced-size liver grafts in paediatric liver transplantation. He contributed greatly to the development of split-liver transplantation and auxiliary liver transplantation, building his techniques on the concepts of liver segmentation, which he helped to establish. Bismuth also developed another international classification system, that of hilar cholangiocarcinoma.

Bismuth received his MD from the University in Paris. Later, he became Head of the Department of Surgery and Director of the HepatoBiliary Center at the Paul Brousse Hospital in Villejuif, France and Professor of Surgery at the Faculty of Medicine at Paris South University. He is a member of the Academie Nationale de Chirurgie and founding President of the French Association of Hepato-Biliary Surgery and Liver Transplantation. Bismuth has received honorary degrees from the Universities of Turin, Porto, Coimbra, and Warsaw and is an honorary member of the American College of Surgeons and the American Surgical Association. Listed on his curriculum vitae is membership of 25 editorial boards.

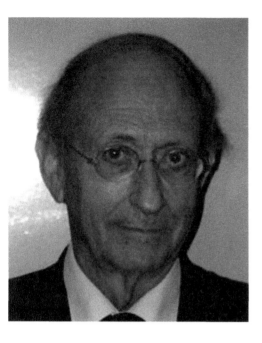

Henri Bismuth. (By kind permission of Professor Henri Bismuth)

References

Bismuth H. Postoperative strictures of the bile duct. In: Blumgart LH. Ed. *Clin Surg Int*. Volume 5. *The Biliary Tract*. Churchill Livingstone, Edinburgh, 1982, pp209–18.

Bismuth H, Houssin D, Castaing D. Major and minor segmentectomies 'réglées' in liver surgery. *World J Surg* 1982;**6**:10–24.

Further reading

Bismuth H. Surgical management of bile duct stricture following laparoscopic cholecystectomy. *Acta Chir Belg* 2003;**103**:140–2.

Bismuth H, Corlette MB. Intrahepatic cholangioenteric anastomosis in carcinoma of the hilus of the liver. *Surg Gynecol Obstet* 1975;**140**:170–8.

Bismuth H, Majno PE. Biliary strictures: classification based on the principles of surgical treatment. *World J Surg* 2001;**25**:1241–4 .

Henri Bismuth Hepatobiliary Institute. http://www.ihb2.org/hb_bio.asp?lang=gb (last accessed 20/5/08).

Boas sign of acute cholecystitis

Boas sign is hyperaesthesia in an area of skin about 2.5 cm to the right of the spinous processes of the 10th to 12th thoracic vertebrae; it is more often loosely referred to as cutaneous hypersensitivity below the right scapula. Boas reported it as a feature of acute cholecystitis in 1902 and Moynihan later endorsed it as a sign of great value (Boas 1902; Moynihan 1904). However, although Gunn and Keddie (1972) reported that 7% of patients undergoing cholecystectomy exhibited cutaneous hyperaesthesia, none of their patients exhibited Boas sign as originally described.

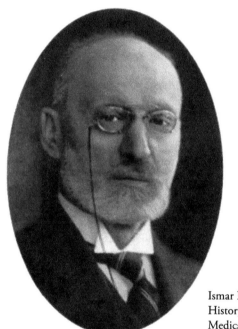

Ismar Isidor Boas. (Courtesy of the Clendening History of Medicine Library, University of Kansas Medical Center)

Ismar Isidor Boas (1858–1938)

Boas worked in Berlin where, despite professional opposition to the concept, he became the first specialist physician in gastrointestinal disease. Among his many achievements, he established the importance of faecal occult bleeding. He founded the German Society of Gastroenterology in 1920 and the first medical journal devoted to gastrointestinal disease (continued today as *Digestion*). With Hitler's rise to power in 1933, Jewish physicians were dismissed from University positions and denied the right to treat non-Jewish patients. After losing his honorary chair at the University of Berlin and the collapse of his medical practice, Boas fled to Vienna in 1936, where he struggled to afford a respectable lifestyle. Three days after the Nazis entered Vienna in March 1938, Boas committed suicide by taking an overdose of a sedative. His son was later killed by the Nazis.

References

Boas I. Beiträge zur Kenntnis der Cholelithiasis. *Münchener medizinische Wochenshrift* 1902;**49**:604–9.

Gunn A, Keddie N. Some clinical observations on patients with gallstones. *Lancet* 1972;**2**:239–41.

Moynihan BGA. *Gall-stones and their Surgical Treatment.* WB Saunders & Co., Philadelphia, 1904, pp116–17.

Further reading

Hoenig LJ, Boyle JD. The life and death of Ismar Boas. *J Clin Gastroenterol* 1988;**10**:16–24.

Strous RD, Edelman MC. Eponyms and the Nazi era: Time to remember and time for change. *Isr Med Assoc J*, 2007;**9**:207–14.

B Budd–Chiari syndrome

Title page for Budd's 1845 text *Diseases of the Liver*

The term 'Budd–Chiari syndrome' is used rather generally today to mean any one of a variety of pathological processes resulting in hepatic venous outflow obstruction at the level of the hepatic veins or retrohepatic vena cava. This results in centrilobular venous congestion and hepatocyte necrosis together with refractory ascites. Potential aetiologies include a vena caval web, neoplastic venous obstruction, trauma and venous thrombosis associated with an underlying thrombophilic disorder. In his book on diseases of the liver published in 1845, Budd reported several cases of hepatic vein phlebitis and thrombosis secondary to hepatic abscess formation (Budd 1845). He observed hepatomegaly, ascites, and the venous collateral circulation consequent on hepatic venous obstruction. He summed up his observations as follows: "[the vein] …becomes closed at that point, and all the branches that feed it, even back to their capillary divisions, become subsequently, and in consequence, choked with fibrine and coagulated blood…".

Hans Chiari's subsequent paper published in 1899 acknowledged the contribution of Budd and others and documented further cases of obliterative phlebitis of large hepatic veins opening into the inferior vena cava (see Budd–Chiari syndrome, p. 38).

George Budd (1808–1882)

George Budd was the third of nine sons, seven of whom became doctors. His father was Samuel Budd, a local surgeon in North Tawton, Devon, England. One of George's brothers, William, became famous for identifying the mechanism of spread

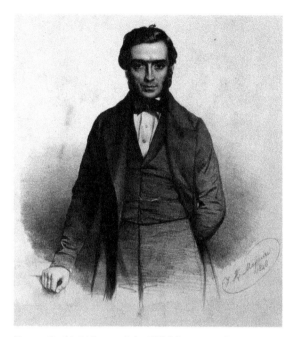

George Budd. Lithograph by TH Maguire 1848.
(V0000864, Courtesy of the Wellcome Library, London)

of typhoid fever. Owing to George's poor health in childhood, he was educated at home. In 1827 he gained a place at Cambridge University, from where he graduated with first class honours in 1831. He then went to Paris, where he studied medicine and pathology before returning to London to enrol as a medical student at the Middlesex Hospital. After qualification he was appointed, at 29 years of age, as Visiting Physician to the Seamen's Hospital Society in London. This society owned the HMS Dreadnought hospital ship, an adapted 104-gun hulk that had served at the Battle of Trafalgar in 1805 and had been released by the Royal Navy to the Seamen's Hospital Society in 1831. It was here that Budd encountered various liver diseases in sailors returning from abroad. During this period, he also carried out research into cholera and published an article on the stethoscope.

In 1840, the same year that he obtained his MD, Budd was appointed as Physician at King's College Hospital, London, where he worked for 23 years. He was a tall, lean man recognised as a skilled and popular teacher and clinical researcher. As well as his book on liver disorders and another *On the Organic Diseases and Functional Disorders of the Stomach* (1855), he wrote numerous medical articles. In one of these, long before the discovery of vitamins, he described three diseases that he correctly considered were due to deficiencies of "accesory food factors": namely, scurvy, keratomalacia, and rickets.

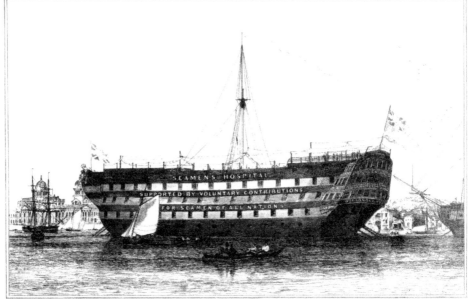

THE DREADNOUGHT, 104 GUNS, UNTIL RECENTLY LYING OFF GREENWICH.

HMS Dreadnought. Engraving circa 1831. (By kind permission of the Seamen's Hospital Society, London)

Budd was a Fellow of the Royal Society (1836) and an honorary Fellow of Caius College, Cambridge (1880). In 1854, at 46 years of age, he married. In 1863, he resigned his position at King's College Hospital and devoted himself to private practice but in 1867 he retired completely from clinical work, largely due to poor health. Thereafter, he took up a rural lifestyle in Devon, enjoying hunting and gardening. He died of pneumonia, at the age of 75 years.

References

Budd G. *Diseases of the Liver*. John Churchill, London, 1845, pp146–8.

Chiari H. Ueber die selbständige Phlebitis obliterans der Hauptstämme der Venae hepaticae als Todesursache. *Beiträge zur Pathologischen Anatomie und Zur Allgemeinen Pathologie* 1899;**26**:1–18.

Further reading

Budd G. Disorders resulting from defective nutrients. *London Med Gaz* 1842;**2**:632–6.

Cook GC. George Budd FRS (1808–1882): pioneer gastroenterologist and hepatologist. *J Med Biog* 1998;**6**:152–9.

Cook GC. History of Medicine: The Seamen's Hospital Society: a progenitor of the tropical institutions. *Postgrad Med J* 1999;**75**:715–17.

Hughes RE. George Budd (1808–1882) and nutritional deficiency diseases. *Med Hist* 1973;**17**:127–35.

McDermott WV, Stone MD, Bothe A, Trey C. Budd–Chiari syndrome. Historical and clinical review with an analysis of surgical corrective procedures. *Am J Surg* 1984;**147**:463–7.

Obituary George Budd MD FRS. *Medical Times and Gazette*, London, 1882;**1**:308.

Obituary Notice of Fellows Deceased. *Proc Roy Soc London* 1882–1883;**34**:i–iii.

Burhenne catheter for extraction of retained biliary calculi

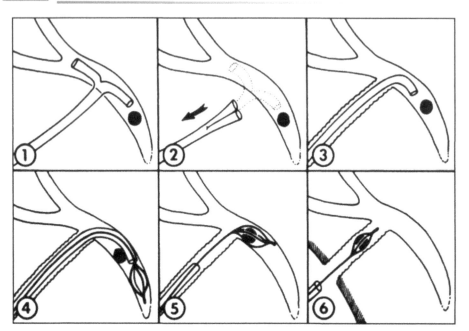

The steps of the Burhenne technique. (1) Repeat T-tube cholangiogram is obtained on the day of stone extraction 4–5 weeks after choledochotomy. (2) After the location of the retained stone has been ascertained, the T-tube is withdrawn. (3) Using the sinus tract of the T-tube, the steerable catheter is guided into the bile duct, and its movable tip is advanced beyond the retained stone. (4) The basket is inserted through the steerable catheter, the catheter is withdrawn and the basket is opened. (5) The open basket is withdrawn in order to engage the stone. The basket is only retracted, never advanced, outside the enclosure of the steerable catheter. (6) The stone is extracted through the drain tract. (From Burhenne HJ. Nonoperative retained biliary tract stone extraction: A new roentgenologic technique. AJR 1973;117:388–99. Reprinted with permission from the American Journal of Roentgenology)

In 1973, Joachim Burhenne, a radiologist in San Francisco, published his technique of percutaneous extraction of retained biliary stones from the common bile duct via the T-tube tract (after cholecystectomy and exploration of the common bile duct). Gallstones had been removed via the T-tube tract by Mondet in Argentina, as early as 1962, using specially designed forceps. Subsequently, others had reported using a Dormia ureteral catheter basket. Burhenne used a novel steerable polyethylene catheter (with an outer diameter of 4.3 mm), which he manipulated under fluoroscopic control and through which a Dormia basket was inserted to extract the stone. In his initial series, 19 of 20 patients were successfully treated without complications. In 1976, Burhenne reported a 5% complication rate and zero mortality associated with the technique in institutions across the United States. In 1980, he reported a personal experience of non-operative biliary stone removal through the T-tube tract in 661 patients; his failure rate was just 5%.

Whilst percutaneous interventional radiological techniques are still widely used in the management of biliary tract disorders, endoscopic retrograde cholangiopancreatography (ERCP) generally provides better access to the common bile duct and does not require a T-tube tract. Endoscopic cannulation of the duodenal papilla was first described by McCune et al in 1968 but ERCP only became widespread after the development and introduction of new duodenoscopes in the 1970s.

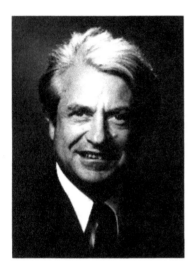

H. Joachim Burhenne. (Courtesy of The Society of Gastrointestinal Radiologists, Houston, Texas, United States)

Joachim Burhenne (1925–1996)

Burhenne was born in Hanover, Germany and graduated from the University of Munich in 1951. On completing residencies in pathology and surgery he moved to the United States, where he trained in radiology at Harvard Medical School and the Peter Bent Brigham Hospital in Boston, Massachusetts. After a research fellowship in England, Burhenne joined the radiology staff at the University of California Medical School in San Francisco in 1960. He moved to Canada in 1978 to become Chairman of the Department of Radiology at the University of British Columbia and Director of Radiology at Vancouver General Hospital. He was the author of more than 250 publications in gastrointestinal radiology, many of which concerned biliary tract interventions.

Burhenne was a founder member of the Society of Gastrointestinal Radiologists and the International Society of Biliary Radiology, becoming President of both. He was described as an enthusiastic, charismatic and ethical leader and was said to be an accomplished skier and violinist. He died of amyotrophic lateral sclerosis.

References

Burhenne HJ. Nonoperative retained biliary tract stone extraction: A new roentgenologic technique. *AJR* 1973;**117**:388–99.

Burhenne HJ. Complications of nonoperative extraction of retained common duct stones. *Am J Surg* 1976;**131**:260–2.

Burhenne HJ. Percutaneous extraction of retained biliary tract stones: 661 patients. *AJR* 1980;**134**:888–98.

McCune WS, Shorb PE, Moscovitz H. Endoscopic cannulation of the ampulla of Vater: a preliminary report. *Ann Surg* 1968;**167**:752–6.

Further reading

Margulis AR. In Memoriam. H Joachim Burhenne, MD, FACR, FRCPC 1925–1996. *Radiology* 1996;**201**:584.

Calot's triangle

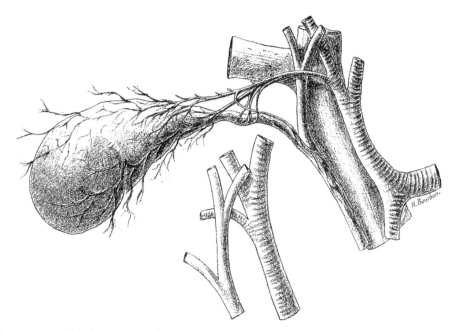

From François Calot's University of Paris doctoral thesis *De la Cholécystectomie*, first published in 1890 by the University and reprinted in 1891. The drawing was made by Henri Bourbon, a medical student. (Courtesy of Dr Stephen J. Greenberg MSLS PhD, Coordinator of Public Services, History of Medicine Division, National Library of Medicine, National Institutes of Health, United States)

In Calot's original description, the superior and inferior sides of this isosceles triangle were the cystic artery and cystic duct, respectively, and the base was formed by the common hepatic duct. Calot commented that the right hepatic artery contributed to the superior border of the triangle for a distance of 3–4 mm in one-third of cases. In many subsequent descriptions of Calot's triangle, the superior border is incorrectly described as the inferior surface of the liver. Although incorrect, it is perhaps a more useful concept when considering the anatomy of cholecystectomy, and supports those who maintain that the triangle should be referred to as the 'hepatobiliary' or 'cystohepatic' triangle.

François Calot (1861–1944)

Calot, a French surgeon, defined the triangle in his doctoral thesis on cholecystectomy *De la Cholécystectomie* published in 1890 in Paris. Calot's thesis focused on the anatomy of the right upper quadrant, particularly in relation to the position of the gall bladder, surgical approaches to it, and the vascular and biliary anatomy in this region. He was concerned with the operation of cholecystectomy, which he probably

23

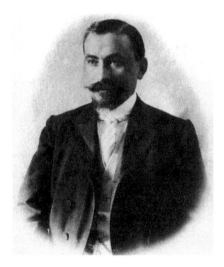 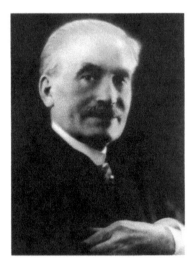

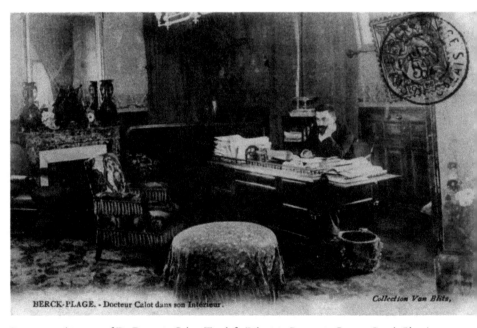

BERCK-PLAGE. - Docteur Calot dans son Intérieur.   Collection Van Blitz,

Portraits and images of Dr François Calot. Top left (Librairie-Papeterie Carnot, Berck-Plage); top right (photograph by G Landrieux); bottom "Docteur Calot dans son Intérieur", Berck-Plage (Van Blitz collection). (By kind courtesy of Dr Christian Morin of the Calot Institute, Berck-sur-Mer, France)

never performed himself, although his chief at the Hôpital Salpêtriére, Louis-Félix Terrier (1837–1908) had undertaken the operation successfully.* Calot insisted that the anatomy of the triangle be clearly delineated before clamps were applied to any structure.

Calot studied medicine at the University of Paris, where he wrote his doctoral thesis. After graduation, he moved to Berck-sur-Mer, a small seaside town in northern France, where he initially worked at several hospitals including the Rothschild Hospital, founded by Baron James de Rothschild (and later sold). Calot's main interest was in orthopaedics, particularly Pott's disease (tuberculosis) of the spine and orthopaedic war wounds. In 1901, he founded his own Institute of Orthopaedics at Berck. This still exists as the Institut Calot. He wrote several orthopaedic textbooks, including *Indispensable Orthopaedics*, which ran to many editions and was translated into five languages.

Calot was a deeply religious man. All four of his brothers were priests. He married and had four daughters, two of whom died in childhood. He retired at 72 years of age and died in his sleep at the age of 83.

* The first clinical cholecystostomy is usually attributed to the American surgeon, John Stough Bobbs (1809–1870), who first successfully performed the operation in July 1867. Similar procedures were reported by the American surgeon and gynaecologist, James Marion Sims (1813–1883), and Theodor Kocher (1841–1917) in 1878. The first cholecystectomy is credited to Carl Langenbuch, a German surgeon working in Berlin in 1882. Just over a century later, in September 1985, the first documented laparoscopic cholecystectomy was performed by Erich Mühe in Germany.

References

Calot F. *De la Cholécystectomie*. Paris, 1890, pp50 & 1891 edition, pp40–3.

Further reading

Brintnall ES. Calot's triangle. *JAMA* 1967;**201**:892.
Loisel P. François Calot, founder of the Orthopedic Institute of Berck. *Hist Sci Med* 2005;**39**:277–83.
Rocko JM, Swan KG, Di Gioia JM. Calot's triangle revisited. *Surg Gynecol Obstet* 1981;**153**:410–14.
Specht MJ. Calot's triangle. *JAMA* 1967;**200**:1186.

C | Cantlie's line

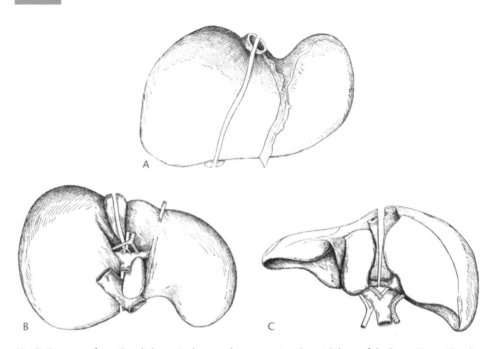

(A–C) Drawings from Cantlie's original paper demonstrating the midplane of the liver. (From Cantlie J. On a new arrangement of the right and left lobes of the liver. *J Anat Physiol* (Lond) 1898;32:iv–ix)

Cantlie had considerable experience of liver pathology, particularly liver abscesses, from his ten years as a surgeon in the Far East. From observations at postmortems, Cantlie realised that the right and left hepatic lobes were functionally distinct. In his 1897 paper, he noted "...a completely separate vascular supply up to the mid-line of the liver...along a line drawn from the centre of the notch for the gall-bladder upon the anterior border of the liver, to the notch for the inferior vena cava at the posterior margin." He followed up this observation with a study of different coloured dyes injected through the right and left portal veins and by weighing the two functional halves of the divided liver, which he found to be similar. He stated that "...surgical interference with the liver will be much more readily tolerated as it approaches that line...". He also speculated that it should be possible to ligate the vessels to the side of the liver in which a tumour was present, leaving the other side to compensate by hypertrophy. The concept of hepatic partitioning based on vascular supply rather than surface morphology was relatively novel at the time and subsequently encouraged the development of safe hepatic resection techniques. Somewhat erroneously, he included the caudate lobe in the left half of the liver.

Cantlie's line has since been designated as the principal plane of the liver, which divides it into left and right halves. The middle hepatic vein is an approximate marker for this plane in imaging studies. The line is unreliable when there are anomalies of the portal vein division (such as a trifurcation or an anterior sectoral trunk originating from the left portal vein).

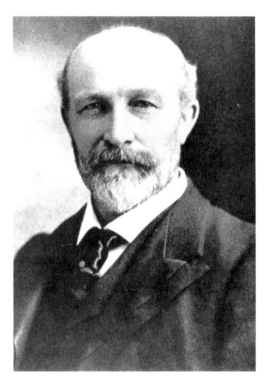

James Cantlie.

James Cantlie (1851–1926)

James Cantlie was born in Banffshire, Scotland and took his first degree in natural sciences at Aberdeen University, before studying clinical medicine at Charing Cross Hospital, London. As a demonstrator of anatomy, he survived 'blood poisoning', which he acquired in the dissecting room. In 1877 he became both a Fellow of the Royal College of Surgeons of England and Assistant Surgeon at Charing Cross Hospital.

In 1885, Cantlie gave several lectures on the subject of the unhealthy air in London, which provoked an uproar in the press and disapproval in some professional circles. Although the controversy did not prevent his promotion to Full Surgeon at Charing Cross it may have been a factor encouraging his move overseas.

He moved to Hong Kong in 1887, where he took over the surgical practice of Patrick Manson (1844–1922) and, together, they founded the Hong Kong College of Medicine for the Chinese (the forerunner of the University of Hong Kong). It was here that the future Chinese leader, Sun Yat-Sen (1866–1925), became one of his pupils. Sun Yat-Sen achieved fame as a revolutionary who orchestrated the overthrow of the Qing dynasty and later became the first President of the Chinese Republic (in 1912). Cantlie was his medical adviser, friend and biographer. He even helped procure the doctor's release when he was kidnapped by Chinese embassy officials whilst living in exile in London.

Cantlie's work in Hong Kong included investigations into leprosy, bubonic plague and various tropical diseases. In 1896 he returned to London, to take up the chair of Applied Anatomy at Charing Cross Hospital Medical School, and it was here that he published his observations on the anatomy of the liver. He established the *Journal of Tropical Medicine* in 1898 and edited this for 25 years. He was among the first faculty members of the London School of Tropical Medicine founded in 1899 and, later, President of the Royal Society of Tropical Medicine and Hygiene. During the early years of the twentieth century and particularly during the First World War (1914–1918), his work centred on the training of ambulance crew and the provision of First Aid. In this, he received considerable support from his wife. During this period he met another future world leader, Mohandas K. Gandhi (1869–1948), who was a member of the Indian Ambulance Unit, which was attached to a contingent of Indian troops fighting alongside the British. Cantlie's interest in First Aid extended back to his years as a junior surgeon at Charing Cross Hospital, when he was a member of the St John's Ambulance Association. He wrote an enduring practical manual for the Association and later one for the British Red Cross Society. Cantlie was knighted for his services to the Red Cross in 1917. He died in 1926.

References

Cantlie J. On a new arrangement of the right and left lobes of the liver. *J Anat Physiol* (Lond) 1898;**32**:iv–ix.

Further reading

Cantlie J. Degeneration amongst Londoners. A lecture. http://www.victorianlondon.org/publications/degeneration.htm (last accessed February 2007).

Chen TS, Chen PS. The accomplishments of Sir James Cantlie. *J Med Biog* 1999;**7**:197–9.

Harris JR. Sir James Cantlie (1851–1926). Founder of the *Journal of Tropical Medicine. J Trop Med* 1973;**76**:185–6.

Ko S, Murakami G, Kanamura T, Sato TJ, Nakajima Y. Cantlie's plane in major variations of the primary portal vein ramification at the porta hepatic: cutting experiment using cadaveric livers. *World J Surg* 2004;**28**:13–18.

Obituary. Sir James Cantlie, KBE, LL.D, FRCS. *Br Med J* 1926;**1**:971–2.

Caroli's disease/syndrome

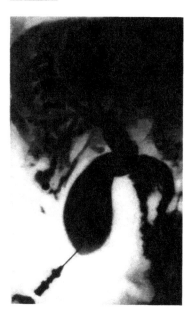

Cholangiogram showing dilatation of the bile duct and peripheral cystic intrahepatic duct dilatation. (From Caroli J, Soupalt R, Kossakowski J, Plocker L, Paradowska M. La dilatation polykystique congenitale des voies biliaires intra-hepatiques. Essai de classification. Semaine des Hôpitaux de Paris 1958;34:488–95 (Fig. 3, p.491). By kind permission of Elsevier Masson SAS)

In 1958, Caroli published two papers describing congenital polycystic dilatation of the intrahepatic bile ducts. In the first, he reported a 13-year-old boy who had a long history of abdominal pain and recurrent cholangitis secondary to diffuse cystic intrahepatic bile duct dilatation (shown in the above Figure). The boy was treated with antibiotics, external biliary drainage and choledochojejunostomy, although it was recognised that this was only palliative treatment. In the second paper, he described a 45-year-old man with recurrent cholangitis secondary to localised cystic dilatation of the left intrahepatic bile ducts. The patient had been treated previously by cholecystectomy and choledochoduodenostomy before presenting again with biliary sepsis. Investigations showed a cavity in the left lobe of the liver and associated biliary stones and debris; he was treated successfully by left hepatectomy.

Two types of congenital polycystic dilatation of the intrahepatic bile ducts are now recognised: the original type (Caroli's disease) and a variety associated with congenital hepatic fibrosis and portal hypertension, usually seen in children (Caroli's syndrome). In both there is segmental saccular communicating intrahepatic bile duct ectasia, frequently accompanied by stone formation, cholangitis and liver abscess formation. Pathology may be limited to a single liver segment or be diffuse. Biliary sepsis or the development of cholangiocarcinoma may be fatal. Caroli's disease and syndrome are the result of a biliary ductal plate malformation, which can be inherited as an autosomal recessive disorder. Both may be associated with a wide range of other conditions such as medullary sponge kidney, infantile polycystic kidney disease and an extrahepatic choledochal cyst.

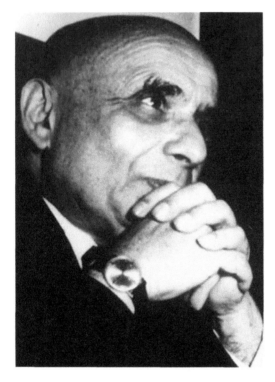

Jacques Caroli.

Jacques Caroli (1902–1979)

Caroli was born near Versailles, France, the son of a physician. He began his medical training in Angers and continued his studies at the Hôtel Dieu Hospital in Paris under the guidance of the renowned biliary tract surgeon, Henri Hartmann (1860–1952). After World War II, Caroli joined the faculty of Saint-Antoine Hospital in Paris, where he was Physician and Chief of Service for 30 years. There he advanced the understanding of a wide range of hepatobiliary disorders. Working with others, including surgeons such as Jacques Hepp and Claude Couinaud, he made important contributions to numerous diagnostic and therapeutic techniques in hepatobiliary disease, notably percutaneous cholangiography, biliary manometry, liver biopsy and laparoscopy. In 1976 he was awarded the prestigious Légion d'Honneur. He was married with children and died in Paris at the age of 77 years.

References

Caroli J, Soupalt R, Kossakowski J, Plocker L, Paradowska M. La dilatation polykystique congenitale des voies biliaires intra-hepatiques. Essai de classification. [Congenital polycystic dilation of the intrahepatic bile ducts; attempt at classification.] *Semaine des Hôpitaux de Paris* 1958a;**34**:488–95.

Further reading

Caroli J, Couinaud C, Soupalt R, Porcher P, Etévé J. Une affection nouvelle, sans doute congénitale, des voies biliaires. La dilatation kystique unilobaire des canaux hépatiques. [A new disease, undoubtedly congenital, of the bile ducts: unilobar cystic dilation of the hepatic ducts.] *Semaine des Hôpitaux de Paris* 1958b;**34**:496–502.

Caroli J. Diseases of the intrahepatic biliary tree. *Clin Gastroenterol* 1973;**2**:147–61.

Haubrich WS. Caroli of Caroli's disease. *Gastroenterology* 2000;**118**:486.

Hepp J. Jacques Caroli and hepatobiliary surgery. *Semaine des Hôpitaux de Paris* 1979;**55**:1879–82.

Paraf A. Jacques Caroli (1902–1979). *La Nouvelle Presse Medicale* 1979;**8**:2493.

C | Carrel patch

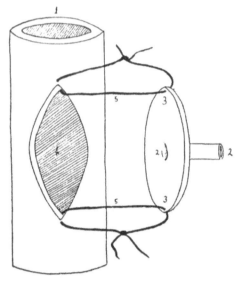

The Carrel patch. A patch from a large donor artery, e.g. the aorta, is used to re-implant a small artery to reduce the risk of thrombosis posed by anastomosis of a small blood vessel. (From Edwards WS, Edwards PD. *Alexis Carrel: Visionary Surgeon*, 1974, p.31, Fig. 7 Patch method of anastomosis. Courtesy of Charles C Thomas Publisher Ltd., Springfield, Illinois)

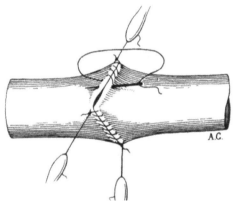

Technique of triangulated vascular anastomosis from Carrel's original 1902 publication in *Lyon Médical*. (Courtesy of the Carrel Collection, Georgetown University, Washington DC)

Carrel's early researches were mainly concerned with vascular anastomosis and organ transplantation. In 1902 he published, in *Lyon Médical*, a triangulation technique for end-to-end anastomosis of blood vessels; it consisted of placing three equidistant stay sutures and an everting running suture between. He also described the Carrel patch technique for reimplantation of small vessels.

Alexis Carrel (1873–1944)

Carrel was born and grew up in France. His father, Alexis Carre-Billiard, died when Carrel was only 4 years old. His mother took on embroidery to supplement her income, providing Carrel with an early introduction to suturing. He gained his

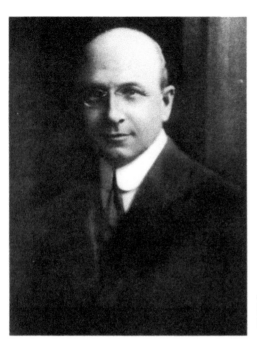

Alexis Carrel. (Courtesy of the Clendening History of Medicine Library, University of Kansas Medical Center)

medical degree from the University of Lyon in 1900 and it was here that he began his experimental research in vascular surgery. His interest in this topic may have been stimulated by the fatal stabbing in Lyon in 1894 of the French President Marie François Sadi Carnot, whose portal vein was severed but could not be repaired.

Carrel was frustrated by his progress in Lyon and in 1904 he journeyed to Canada with the idea of raising cattle. However, he soon moved to the University of Chicago, where he worked with the American physiologist, Charles Guthrie. Together, they transplanted kidneys, thyroids and ovaries in experimental animals. He took up a position at the Rockefeller Institute for Medical Research in New York two years later. Carrel's pioneering work in vascular anastomotic techniques was a major surgical achievement. This, together with his research into cold storage of blood vessels and organ transplantation, earned him the Nobel Prize in Physiology or Medicine in 1912, at just 39 years of age. He used the prize money to buy the tiny island of Saint-Gildas, off the coast of Brittany in France. This became a beloved summer retreat for Carrel and his wife, a young, widowed nurse whom he married in 1913; they had no children.

Whilst serving in the French Army during World War I, he developed, with the chemist Henry Dakin, a method of wound irrigation using the antiseptic sodium hypochlorite, a significant advance in pre-antibiotic wound care. For this work, he was awarded the French Légion d'Honneur. In 1917, he returned to the Rockefeller Institute to direct a war demonstration hospital.

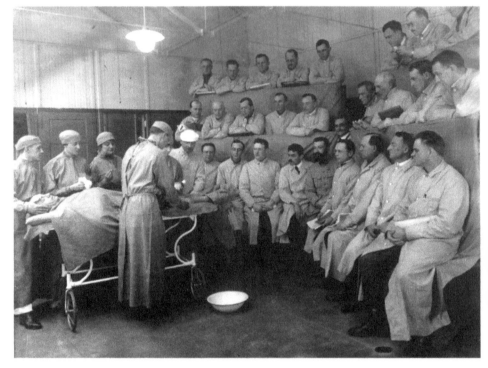

Alexis Carrel (in white cap) demonstrating at a Rockefeller Institute War Demonstration Hospital during World War I. (Courtesy of The Granger Collection, New York [0004759])

His subsequent research focused on tissue and organ culture. Together with the aviator Charles A. Lindbergh, he devised a perfusion pump that could maintain the viability of animal organs outside the body. In 1938 they published *The Culture of Organs*. However, his famous experiment of maintaining an embryonic chick's heart tissue *in vitro* for more than 20 years was never replicated, probably because it was reliant on the introduction of fresh cells with the nutrient solution.

Carrel wrote several other books, including *Reflections on Life* (1952) and a bestseller, *Man, the Unknown* (1935), in which he expressed controversial and offensive views about the role of eugenics and euthanasia, believing in the 'perpetuation of the strong'. Carrel retired from the Rockefeller Institute in 1939. During World War II he lived in France and was Director of the Foundation for the Study of Human Problems under the Vichy regime. After the war he was accused of being a Nazi collaborator, partly because of his eugenic theories. He died from ischaemic heart disease in Paris in 1944 and was buried in the Chapel of St Yves near his house on Saint-Gildas. Concerns about Carrel's elitist and racist views persist to this day – his name was removed from streets in French cities in the 1990s and in 1996, the University of Lyon renamed its school of medicine after René Laennec, inventor of the stethoscope (see Laennec p. 105).

Two of his books, *The Prayer* (1948) and *Voyage to Lourdes* (1949), were published posthumously. He received honorary doctorates from universities in the United States and Europe, was featured twice on the cover of *TIME* magazine (16 September 1935 and, with Charles A. Lindbergh, 13 June 1938), and was commemorated on a Swedish postage stamp (1972) and by the naming of a lunar crater after him (1979). A collection of Alexis Carrel's works can be found in the Georgetown University Library, Washington, DC.

References

Carrel A. Anastomose bout à bout de la jugulaire et de la carotide primitive. *Lyon Médical* 1902;**99**:114.

Carrel A. La technique opératoire des anastomoses vasculaires et la transplantation des viscères. *Lyon Médical* 1902;**98**:859–64.

Edwards WS, Edwards PD. *Alexis Carrel: Visionary Surgeon.* Charles C. Thomas Publisher Ltd., Springfield, Illinois, 1974.

Further reading

Alexis Carrel. The Nobel Prize in Physiology or Medicine 1912. Nobelprize.org (Last accessed October 2008).

Anon. Industry to Profit by Surgery of War. *New York Times* 16 July, 1917.

Carrel A. On the permanent life of tissues outside of the organism. *J Exp Med* 1912;**15**:516–28.

Carrel A, Guthrie CC. Successful transplantation of both kidneys from a dog into a bitch with removal of both normal kidneys from the latter. *Science* 1906;**23**:394–5.

Dutkowski P, de Rougemont O, Clavien PA. Alexis Carrel: Genius, innovator and ideologist. *Am J Transpl* 2008;**8**:1998–2003.

Enersen OD. Editor: whonamedit.com, a biographical dictionary of medical eponyms. http://www.whonamedit.com/doctor.cfm/445.html (Last accessed November 2008).

Langer RM, Kahan BD. Alexis Carrel's legacy: visionary of vascular surgery and organ transplantation. *Transplant Proc* 2002;**34**:1061–5.

Malinin TI. *Surgery and life: the extraordinary career of Alexis Carrel.* Harcourt Brace Jovanovich, New York, 1979.

Sade RM. Transplantation at 100 years: Alexis Carrel, Pioneer Surgeon. *Ann Thorac Surg* 2005;**80**:2415–18.

C Charcot's intermittent hepatic fever/ Charcot's triad

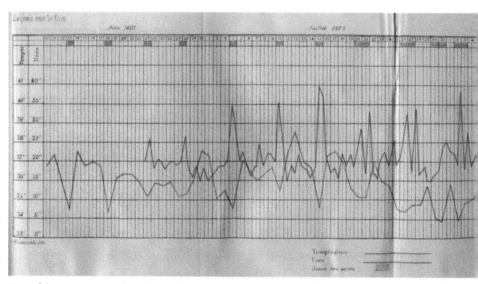

Part of the temperature chart from Charcot's original description of intermittent hepatic fever. This was recorded during a period of 3 months from a 68-year-old man who at autopsy was found to have bile duct obstruction from a gallstone. Bouts of high fever up to 41°C occurred every 5–6 days (red line). The green line is the patient's urea level. (From Charcot JM. Leçons sur les Maladies du Foie des Voies Biliaires et des Reins. Bourneville et Sevestre, Paris, 1877, Plate IV, p.358)

Charcot's intermittent hepatic fever is associated with common bile duct obstruction. This is usually but not always due to cholelithiasis with cholangitis; in Charcot's time, the condition was frequently fatal. Charcot attributed the fever to a 'morbid pyrogenic poison' resulting from an alteration of the bile since evidence of suppurative cholangitis was not always found in such cases.

Charcot's triad consists of jaundice, fever with rigors and right upper quadrant abdominal pain, and is typically associated with cholangitis secondary to choledocholithiasis. Reynolds' pentad is a combination of Charcot's triad with hypotension and an altered mental state; it is named after Benedict M. Reynolds, a New York surgeon who described it in 1959 (Reynolds 1959).

Jean Martin Charcot (1825–1893)

The son of a Paris coachbuilder, Charcot and his three brothers were sent to school for one year on the understanding that the boy who received the best report would be allowed to study a learned profession. He won and chose medicine.

Charcot was appointed as Physician to the Paris hospital of Salpêtrière in 1862, where he later became the first Professor of Neurology (1882), a chair created by the French Parliament. His neurology clinics became legendary, not least because of his charisma and somewhat theatrical case presentations. He was a talented artist and well read in the classics, which he frequently quoted in his lectures. Charcot also

C

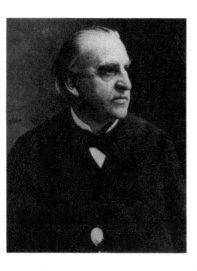

Jean Martin Charcot. (Courtesy of the Université P. & M. Curie, Service Commun de la Documentation Médicale, Bibliothèque Charcot, Hôpital de la Salpêtrière, Paris)

had a keen interest in music, and was particularly fond of Beethoven. He married an heiress and lived in style in the Boulevard Saint-Germain in Paris, where he kept several pets, including a Brazilian monkey called Rosalie, a gift from the Brazilian Emperor.

Charcot was an outstanding neurologist and described multiple sclerosis, the lightning pains of tabes dorsalis, the joint destruction associated with severe neuropathy (Charcot's joints), peroneal muscular atrophy and intermittent claudication. Even more dramatic, though less significant, were his descriptions of hysteria and hypnotism, which had a significant influence on Sigmund Freud.

Charcot was said to have a strong physical resemblance to Napoleon and, like him, he did not tolerate contradiction. He died suddenly from ischaemic heart disease at 68 years of age. A commemorative stamp was issued in France in his honour in 1960.

References

Charcot JM. *Leçons sur les Maladies du Foie des Voies Biliaires et des Reins*. Bourneville et Sevestre, Paris, 1877, pp146–56, 176–85, 194–8.

Reynolds BM, Dargan EL. Acute obstructive cholangitis: a distinct clinical syndrome. *Ann Surg* 1959;**150**:299–303.

Further reading

Ellis H. *Bailey and Bishop's Notable Names in Medicine and Surgery*. 4th edition. H.K.Lewis & Co. Ltd, London, 1983, pp28–30.

Guillain G. *JM Charcot 1825–1893: His life – His work*. Paul B. Hoeber, New York, 1959.

Morgenstern L. Jean-Martin Charcot and 'Charcot's Fever'. *New Engl J Med* 1959;**261**:36–7.

Teive HA, Arruda WO, Werneck LC. Rosalie: the Brazilian female monkey of Charcot. *Arq Neuropsiquiatr* 2005;**63**:707–8.

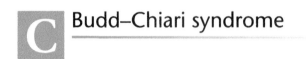

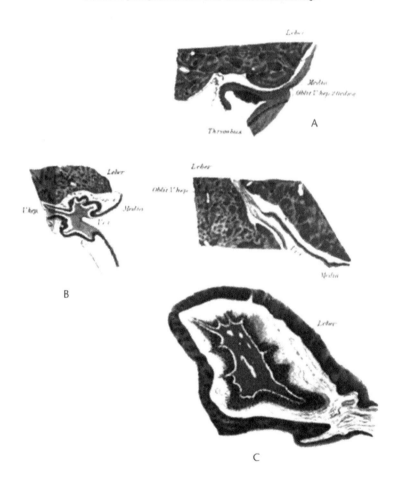

Ueber die selbständige Phlebitis obliterans der Hauptstämme der Venae hepaticae als Todesursache.¹⁾

Von

Dr. H. Chiari,

Professor der pathologischen Anatomie an der deutschen Universität in Prag.

Illustrations from Chiari H. Ueber die selbständige Phlebitis obliterans der Hauptstämme der Venae hepaticae als Todesursache. Beiträge zur Pathologischen Anatomie und Zur Allgemeinen Pathologie 1899;26:1–18. Top (**A**): Cross-sectional view of hepatic vein with intimal and parietal thrombosis and obliteration in the termination of a second order hepatic vein. Middle (**B**). Left: Obliteration of the ostium of the hepatic vein entering the inferior vena cava. Right: Obliteration of the ostia of small hepatic veins from the inferior vena cava. Bottom (**C**): Obliteration of hepatic vein 2 cm away from the entry into the inferior vena cava. (By kind permission of the Royal Society of Medicine)

38

C

Budd–Chiari syndrome is the term used today to refer to the constellation of features resulting from venous outflow obstruction of the liver at the level of the hepatic veins or retrohepatic vena cava. Both acute and chronic presentations are now recognised, the latter progressing to cirrhosis. Hans Chiari's paper published in 1899 acknowledged the contribution of George Budd (1808–1882) (see Budd–Chiari p. 16) and others and included descriptions of new cases of obliterative phlebitis affecting large hepatic veins opening into the inferior vena cava (Chiari 1899).

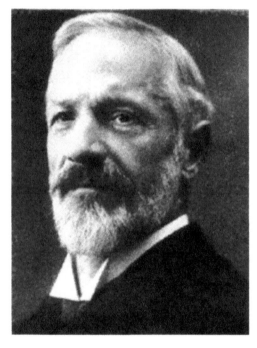

Hans Chiari.

Hans Chiari (1851–1916)

Hans Chiari was born in Vienna in 1851, the son of a famous obstetrician and gynaecologist, Johann Chiari, who described postpartum galactorrhoea and amenorrhoea secondary to pituitary dysfunction. Hans studied medicine in Vienna, where he was an assistant to the famous Austrian pathologist, Carl von Rokitansky (1804–1878) (see Rokitansky–Aschoff sinus p. 171). After graduation in 1875, Chiari was appointed as a pathological anatomist in Vienna. Subsequently, he became professor of pathology at the German University in Prague and later, in 1906, he took up the Chair in Pathology at Strasbourg.

From his vast knowledge gained from systematic postmortem examinations, he published extensively on a wide range of subjects in pathology including chorionic carcinoma, syringomyelia, pancreatitis, and congenital cardiac malformations. Chiari was possibly the first to postulate that pancreatitis was due to pancreatic autodigestion and not due to the spread of inflammation from the stomach and duodenum, as had been previously thought. However, he is best remembered for the Arnold–Chiari malformation, which he described in 1891 (Chiari 1891). This is a malformation in which the inferior cerebellum and brainstem protrude through the foramen magnum into the vertebral canal, typically in association with congenital hydrocephalus. As with his description of hepatic venous thrombophlebitis, he was careful to acknowledge the contributions of others (in this case that of Arnold, whose name was subsequently added to the malformation in 1907 by two of his students who reported additional cases).

Chiari was renowned for his meticulous attention to detail but tended to be irascible. He became so irritated if his students prepared tissue sections poorly that he would rap their knuckles. He died suddenly from a throat infection at the age of 64 years.

References

Chiari H. Üeber die selbständige Phlebitis obliterans der Hauptstämme der Venae hepaticae als Todesursache. *Beiträge zur Pathologischen Anatomie und Zur Allgemeinen Pathologie* 1899;**26**:1–18.

Chiari H. Üeber Veränderungen des Kleinhirns infolge von Hydrocephalie des Grosshirns. *Deutsche Medicinische Wochenschrift* 1891;**17**:1172–5.

Further reading

Budd G. *On Diseases of the Liver*. John Churchill, London, 1845, pp146–8.

Chiari H. Ueber die Selbstverdauung des menschlichen Pankreas. *Z Heilk* 1896;**17**:69–96.

Loukas M, Noordeh N, Shoja MM, Pugh J, Oakes WJ, Tubbs RS. Hans Chiari (1851–1916). *Childs Nerv Syst* 2008;**24**:407–9.

O'Reilly DA, Kingsnorth AN. A brief history of pancreatitis. *J Roy Soc Med* 2001;**94**:130–2.

Pearce JMS. Arnold Chiari, or 'Cruveilhier Cleland Chiari' malformation. *J Neurol Neurosurg Psychiatry* 2000;**68**:13.

C Child's classification of severity of liver disease

Child and Turcotte first proposed the classification in 1964 (Child and Turcotte 1964). The aim was to stratify patients with cirrhosis according to their hepatic functional reserve. The original classification divided patients into three groups: A, B and C:

Clinical and laboratory classification of patients with cirrhosis in terms of hepatic functional reserve

Group designation	A Minimal	B Moderate	C Advanced
Serum bilirubin (mg%)	Below 2.0	2.0–3.0	Over 3.0
Serum albumin (g%)	Over 3.5	3.0–3.5	Under 3.0
Ascites	None	Easily controlled	Poorly controlled
Neurological disorder	None	Minimal	Advanced, 'coma'
Nutrition	Excellent	Good	Poor, 'wasting'

(From Child CG 3rd, Turcotte JG. Surgery and portal hypertension. In: Child CG 3rd, Dunphy JE, eds. *Major Problems in Clinical Surgery.* Volume 1: The Liver and Portal Hypertension. W B Saunders, Philadelphia, 1964, p.50)

Child and Turcotte found that the classification could be used to select patients for elective portosystemic shunting since functional hepatic reserve provided a more accurate prediction of postoperative morbidity and mortality than age, sex or type of cirrhosis.

The classification was modified into a scoring system by Pugh* and colleagues in 1973 (Pugh et al 1973). Child's criterion of nutritional status was replaced with a measure of prolongation of the prothrombin time. The Child–Pugh score was assessed as follows:

Grading of severity of liver disease

Clinical and biochemical measurements	Points scored for increasing abnormality		
	1	2	3
Encephalopathy (grade)	None	1 and 2	3 and 4
Ascites	Absent	Slight	Moderate
Bilirubin (mg%)*	1–2	2–3	> 3
Albumin (g%)	3.5	2.8–3.5	< 2.8
Prothrombin time (sec. prolonged)	1–4	4–6	> 6

*Bilirubin levels are higher for primary biliary cirrhosis. (From Pugh RNH, Murray-Lyon IM, Dawson JL, Pietroni MC, Williams R. Transection of the oesophagus for bleeding oesophageal varices. *Br J Surg* 1973;60:647)

Patents with cirrhosis and portal hypertension who had total scores of 5–6 were grade A (good operative risk); 7–9 grade B (moderate); and 10–15 grade C (poor

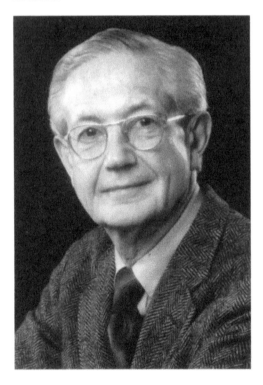

Charles G. Child 3rd. (Courtesy of the department of Surgery, Center for Surgery Emeritus Faculty, University of Michigan Medical School)

operative risk). The score also proved to be of prognostic value in patients with chronic liver disease.

˙Nicholas Pugh (1946–), research physician and clinical epidemiologist is currently a public health physician in Walsall, UK.

Charles Gardner Child 3rd (1908–1991)

Charles Gardner Child 3rd graduated from Yale University in 1930 and from Cornell University Medical College in 1934. He initially worked at New York Hospital. From 1953–1958 he was Chairman of the department of Surgery at Tufts University and from 1959–1974 Chairman of the department of Surgery at the University of Michigan. In 1977 he moved to Emory University in Atlanta, Georgia, where he was Professor of Surgery.

His major contributions were in surgery of the pancreas and portal hypertension. He wrote several books on portal hypertension.

Child was a member of the National Academy of Sciences and held several prestigious appointments including Chairman of the American Board of Surgery and committee positions within the American Surgical Association. He was the founding Editor of the *Journal of Surgical Research*. Charles Child was married with five children. He died in his sleep at his home in Atlanta.

References

Child CG 3rd, Turcotte JG. Surgery and portal hypertension. In: Child CG 3rd, Dunphy JE, eds. *Major Problems in Clinical Surgery.* Volume 1: *The Liver and Portal Hypertension.* W B Saunders, Philadelphia, 1964, pp1–85.

Pugh RNH, Murray-Lyon IM, Dawson JL, Pietroni MC, Williams R. Transection of the oesophagus for bleeding oesophageal varices. *Br J Surg* 1973;**60**:646–9.

Further reading

Turcotte JG. In memoriam. Charles Gardner Child 3rd 1908–1991. *Surgery* 1992;111:601.

C | Couinaud's liver segments

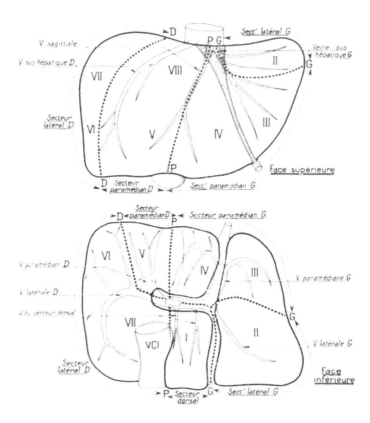

Couinaud's scheme for segmental anatomy of the liver. The liver segments are numbered clockwise with Roman numerals. Segment I is the caudate lobe. The hepatic veins are shown in the upper figure and the portal vein divisions in the lower figure. (From Couinaud C. Le Foie: Études Anatomiques et Chirurgicales. Masson & Co., Paris, 1957, p.533)

Couinaud first reported his observations on intrahepatic vascular and biliary anatomy in 1952 (Couinaud 1952). Two years later he published an account of liver segmental anatomy, which formed the basis for his seminal 1957 text (Couinaud 1957). Using the more consistent branching pattern of the portal vein, eight liver segments were defined beginning with the caudate lobe (segment I); these were numbered progressively in a clockwise manner. Segments were organised into four sectors (right lateral, right paramedian, left paramedian and left lateral) by the three main hepatic veins located in the fissures or planes between portal sectors. Each sector was generally supplied by one vasculobiliary sheath but the segmental pattern was more variable. The caudate lobe was difficult to classify and, at various times, Couinaud referred to it as segment I, segment IX, and more latterly as the dorsal or posterior sector of the liver.

C

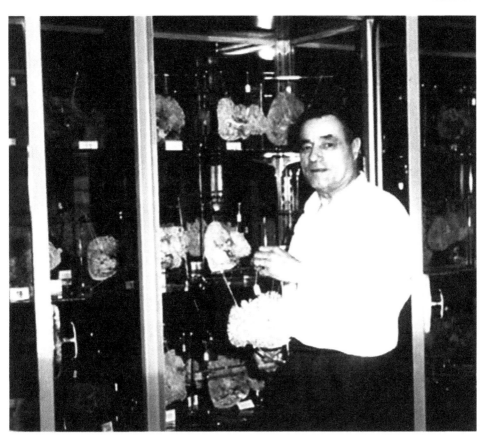

Claude Couinaud working with his collection of liver casts at the School of Medicine in Paris, 1988. (Reproduced with permission from Sutherland F, Harris J. Claude Couinaud. A passion for the liver. Arch Surg 2002;137:1305–10, Fig 1, p.1305. Copyright © 2002 American Medical Association. All rights reserved)

Claude Couinaud (1922–)

Born at Neuilly-sur-Seine, Couinaud grew up in Argentan, France and studied medicine at the École de Medicine de Paris, entering his surgical residency in 1946. He graduated in 1951, winning the gold medal in the process, and then visited Philip Allison (1907–1974) in Leeds, England to investigate bronchopulmonary anatomy before returning to Paris to study the anatomy of the liver under the direction of André Delmas. He reviewed the earlier works of Hugo Rex and others and insisted on naming the vasculobiliary sheaths of the liver after Johannus Walaeus (1604–1649), whose work predated that of Francis Glisson (1597–1677) by two years.

45

Couinaud's anatomic studies of the liver were facilitated by a corrosion cast technique using polyvinyl acetone injected into the portal triad structures. He made precise drawings of each cast and noted a consistent segmental pattern, which was to provide the basis for his classification of segmental anatomy.

In 1952, Couinaud resumed clinical practice as chief resident but continued with his anatomical studies. In addition to his definitive description of liver segmental anatomy in 1954. Couinaud made several other major contributions to the surgical anatomy of the liver:

1. Vasculobiliary (Glissonian) sheaths: Couinaud noted that these condensations of fibrous tissue were organised into four plates: the gall bladder bed plate; the hilar plate; the umbilical plate (in the umbilical fissure), and the plate of Arantius (covering the ductus venosus). The portal triad structures enter the liver through the hilar and umbilical plates, gaining a common fibrous sheath in the process. Couinaud recommended vascular control during major hepatic resection by ligating the relevant Glissonian pedicle ('controlled' hepatectomy).
2. He identified a relatively avascular plane between the retrohepatic vena cava and the liver, a space that can be exploited in liver resections.
3. Couinaud's understanding of liver plate anatomy led him to suggest that the hilar plate could be lowered by dissecting above it within segment IV, thereby improving access to the well-vascularised extrahepatic segment of the left hilar duct. A high wide hepaticojejunostomy could then be performed as described by Jacques Hepp and Claude Couinaud in 1956. This has proved to be an enduring biliary bypass procedure for hilar duct strictures.

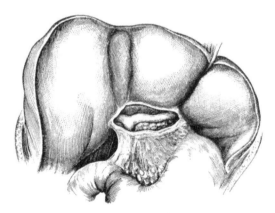

Lowering the hilar plate in preparation for a left hepatic duct biliary bypass (Reprinted with permission from Hepp J, Couinaud C. L'abord et l'utilisation du canal hépatiques gauche dans les reparations de la voie biliaire principale. La Presse Médicale 1956;64:947, Fig. 1. © Elsevier Masson)

4. He demonstrated that a segment III biliary bypass is sometimes possible when access to the proximal left hepatic duct is not. However, variations in segment II, III and IV biliary anatomy in up to one-third of individuals limits the application of this technique.
5. Finally, he made several contributions to the anatomy of surgical techniques in split-liver and live-related liver transplantation.

Couinaud published his famous book *Le Foie: Études Anatomiques et Chirurgicales* in 1957; this included not only descriptive anatomy of the liver and surgical approaches but also details of comparative and developmental anatomy. In addition, he self-published two other books: *Surgical Anatomy of the Liver Revisited* and *Tell Me More About Liver Anatomy* (Couinaud 1989, 1999). Other research interests included the prevention of venous thromboembolism with heparin, zinc deficiency and pressure sores in the elderly.

From 1958 until his retirement in 1975, Couinaud worked at the Saint Louis Hospital in Paris. After his retirement, he continued to work on his liver casts housed at the University of Paris Faculty of Medicine. He received the International Medal of Surgery ('Lannelongue') from the Academie Française de Chirurgie in 1992, the Gold Medal from Nagoya University in Japan in 1993, and the Theresian medal of the University of Pavia in Italy in 1995.

References

Couinaud C. Distribution intraparenchymateuse des vaisseaux hepatiques et des voles biliaires, 2:foie droite. *Comptes Rendus de l Association des Anatomistes* 1952;**39**:318–23.

Couinaud C. *Le Foie: Études Anatomiques et Chirurgicales.* Masson Publishing USA Inc, New York, 1957, p.533

Couinaud C. Lobes et segments hepatiques: Notes sur l'architecture anatomique et chirurgicale de foie. *Presse Med* 1954;**62**:709–12.

Couinaud C. *Surgical Anatomy of the Liver Revisited.* Paris, 1989.

Couinaud C. *Tell me more about Liver Anatomy.* Paris, 1999.

Hepp J, Couinaud C. L'abord et l'utilisation du canal hépatiques gauche dans les reparations de la voie biliaire principale. *Presse Med* 1956;**64**:947–8.

Sutherland F, Harris J. Claude Couinaud. A passion for the liver. *Arch Surg* 2002;**137**:1305–10.

Further reading

Abdalla EK, Vauthey JN, Couinaud C. The caudate lobe of the liver: implications of embryology and anatomy for surgery. *Surg Oncol Clin N Am* 2002;**11**:835–48.

Couinaud C. Les hépato-cholangiostomies digestives. *Presse Med* 1953;**61**:468–70.

Couinaud C. Les envelopes vasculo-biliaires du foie ou capsule de Glisson: leur interet dans la Chirurgie vesiculaire, les resections hepatiques et l'abord du hile du foie. *Lyon Chir* 1954;**49**:589–607.

Couinaud's liver segments

Couinaud C. Exposure of the left hepatic duct through the hilum or in the umbilical of the liver: anatomic limitations. *Surgery* 1989;**105**:21–7.

Couinaud C. A scandal: segment IV and liver transplantation. *J Chir (Paris)*1993;**130**:443–6.

Couinaud C. Dorsal sector of the liver. *Chirurgie* 1998;**123**:8–15.

Couinaud C. Liver anatomy: Portal (and suprahepatic) or biliary segmentation. *Dig Surg* 1999;**16**:459–67.

Couinaud C, Houssin D. *Controlled Partition of the Liver for Transplantation: Anatomical Limitations.* Paris, 1991.

Soupault R, Couinaud C. Sur un procede nouveau de derivation biliaire intrahepatique: les cholangio-jejunostomies gauches sans sacrifice hepatique. *Presse Med* 1957;**65**:1157–9.

Walaeus J. Epistolae duae de motu chilli et sanguinis ad Thomam Bartholeum. In: Thomas Bartholeus. *Anatomia Lugd.* Bataviae (Leyden), the Netherlands. Fransciscus Hackius, 1640.

Courvoisier's Law

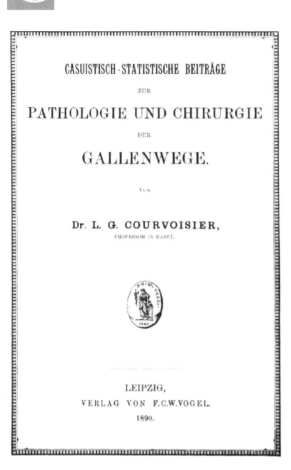

CASUISTISCH-STATISTISCHE BEITRÄGE

ZUR

PATHOLOGIE UND CHIRURGIE

DER

GALLENWEGE.

VON

Dr. L. G. COURVOISIER,

PROFESSOR IN BASEL.

LEIPZIG,
VERLAG VON F.C.W.VOGEL.
1890.

Title page from Courvoisier's 1890 monograph. (Courtesy of Goettingen State and University Library)

Courvoisier's Law states that: "with obstruction of the common duct by a stone, dilatation [of the gall bladder] is rare. With obstruction from other kinds, distension is the rule." This is often expressed as: 'If in the presence of jaundice the gall bladder is palpable, then the jaundice is unlikely to be due to a stone'. The 'law' is based on the probability that the gall bladder is usually thickened and fibrotic and does not distend if the common bile duct is obstructed by a stone. Common bile duct obstruction from other causes, typically carcinoma of the head of the pancreas, is usually associated with a normal distensible gall bladder. The law was first enunciated by Courvoisier in his monograph *The Pathology and Surgery of the Biliary Tract* published in 1890 (Courvoisier 1890). He appropriately described it as a useful sign in differential diagnosis rather than a law since it was not an invariable finding. Indeed, Courvoisier found dilatation of the gall bladder in 17 (20%) of 87 patients with calculous obstruction of the common bile duct but in only two of these was the gall bladder markedly enlarged. This compared to 92% of 100 patients with

49

other causes of common bile duct obstruction (extrinsic compression, tumours and strictures), many of whom had a markedly enlarged gall bladder. He concluded that gall bladder dilatation seldom occurs when the common bile duct is obstructed by a stone. Confirmation of these findings by Mayo Robson, Moynihan and others soon led to the observation being referred to as Courvoisier's Law.

The general validity of Courvoisier's sign has since been affirmed by many authors. However, recent studies have suggested it is less clear cut, perhaps because Courvoisier's observations were based on more advanced cases of obstructive jaundice than seen today. Furthermore, the pathophysiological basis of the clinical sign has been questioned. Chung (1983) found that malignant obstruction of the common bile duct was associated with higher intraductal pressures of longer duration than obstruction due to stones, but there was no difference in the distensibility of freshly excised gall bladders in such cases.

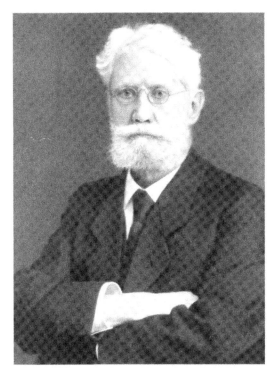

Ludwig G. Courvoisier. (Courtesy of the Deutsches Entomologisches Institut, Müncheberg, Germany)

Ludwig Georg Courvoisier (1843–1918)

Courvoisier was born in Basel, Switzerland. His father was a merchant and his mother the daughter of an English clergyman. Despite an interruption to his medical studies by a near-fatal bout of typhoid (typhus in some accounts), he obtained his medical degree from the University of Basel in 1868, winning a prize for his thesis on the histology of the sympathetic nervous system. He undertook postgraduate studies in London with Sir Thomas Spencer Wells and in Vienna with Theodor Billroth and Vincenz Czerny. During the Franco–Prussian war, he served in a military hospital at Karlsruhe in Germany. After the war he worked in the Diakonissenspital (Deaconess Hospital) in Riehen, a small town on the German–Swiss border, and subsequently developed a successful private practice in Basel. In 1888, the University of Basle conferred on him the title of Extraordinary Professor of Surgery.

Courvoisier's main interest was the biliary tract. He was among the first to describe the removal of a gallstone from the common bile duct. In his monograph of 1890 he discussed common bile duct obstruction from various causes.

In his spare time, Courvoisier was an avid natural historian, pursuing his childhood hobbies of collecting butterflies and studying plants. He published numerous papers on entomology. He died from pneumonia at 75 years of age and bequeathed his collection of butterflies to the Natural History Museum in Basel and his herbarium to the Botanical Institute of Basel.

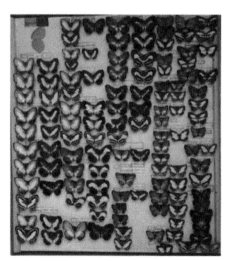 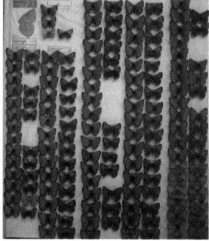

Example drawers from Courvoisier's butterfly collection. (Courtesy of Dr Daniel Burckhardt of the Naturhistorisches Museum, Basel, Switzerland)

References

Chung RS. Pathogenesis of the 'Courvoisier gallbladder'. *Dig Dis Sci* 1983;**28**:33–8.

Courvoisier LG. *Casuistisch-Statistische Beiträge zur Pathologie und Chirurgie der Gallenwege.* FCW Vogel, Leipzig, 1890, pp57–9.

Mayo Robson AW. *On gall-stones and their treatment.* Cassell & Co., London, 1892.

Moynihan BGA. *Gall-stones and their surgical treatment.* WB Saunders & Co, Philadelphia, 1904, pp128–32.

51

Courvoisier's Law

Further reading

Anon. Ludwig Courvoisier (1843–1918) Courvoisier's sign. *JAMA* 1968;**204**:165.

Ellis H. *Bailey and Bishop's Notable Names in Medicine and Surgery.* 4th edition. H.K.Lewis & Co. Ltd, London, 1983, pp44–7.

Morgenstern L. Luwig G. Courvoisier and Courvoisier's Law. *Surg Gynecol Obstet* 1960;**110**:383–4.

Veillon E. Professor Dr med L G Courvoisier. *Correspondenzblatt für Schweizer Ärzte*, Basel, 1918;**48**:1314–19.

Verghese A, Dison C, Berk SL. Courvoisier's 'Law' – an eponym in evolution. *Am J Gastroenterol* 1987;**82**:248–50.

Viteri AL. Courvoisier's law and evaluation of the jaundiced patient. *Tex Med* 1980;**76**:60–1.

Wood M. Eponyms in biliary tract surgery. *Am J Surg* 1979;**138**:746–54.

C Cullen's sign

Cullen's sign refers to bluish-black skin discolouration of the periumbilical region due to the tracking of retroperitoneal blood. Cullen first described the sign in 1918 in a 38-year-old woman with a ruptured ectopic pregnancy (Cullen 1989). These days, the sign is usually associated with acute haemorrhagic pancreatitis, although it is rarely seen. Extravasated blood and inflammatory fluid may reach the periumbilical region from the retroperitoneum either via the lesser omentum and falciform ligament or via the pararenal spaces and abdominal wall. Other causes of extraperitoneal bleeding such as a rectus sheath haematoma occasionally produce a similar effect.

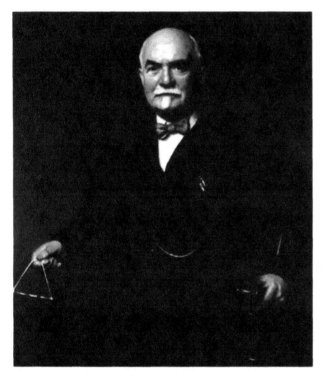

Thomas Stephen Cullen. (By Thomas C. Corner, oil on canvas, 1907, Courtesy of The Alan Mason Chesney Medical Archives of The Johns Hopkins Medical Institutions, photograph by Aaron Levin)

Thomas Stephen Cullen (1868–1953)

Cullen was Professor of Gynecology at Johns Hopkins Hospital in Baltimore, MD from 1919. A Canadian by birth, he obtained his medical degree from the University of Toronto in 1890. Between 1893 and 1896 he took charge of gynaeclogical pathology at Johns Hopkins after a residency position that he had been promised fell through. He later recounted that this was the making of his career. Subsequently, he progressed through the ranks in gynaecology, developing an international reputation in the process. Cullen's numerous publications included four major texts, all of which were richly illustrated by his close friend, the medical artist, Max Brödel. As   53 a result of this experience, he became a keen advocate of art in medicine. Following a cholecystectomy for gallstone disease in 1923, Brödel presented Cullen with a framed picture of his name and the date of the operation made from his gallstones!

References

Cullen TS. A new sign in ruptured extrauterine pregnancy. *Am J Obstet* 1918;**78**:457.

Further reading

Harris S, Naina HVK. Cullen's sign revisited. *Am J Med* 2008;**121**:682–3.

Robinson J. *Tom Cullen of Baltimore*. Oxford University Press, London, 1949.

Young RH. History of gynecological pathology. I. Dr Thomas S. Cullen. *Int J Gynecol Pathol* 1996;**15**:181–6.

Deaver retractor

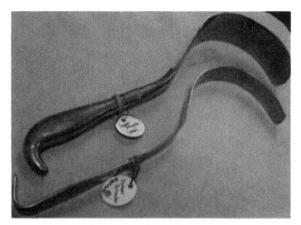

The Deaver retractor. (Courtesy of Daniel Peters, Leander, Texas, USA)

The Deaver retractor was designed for retracting the liver during cholecystectomy. Deaver did not allow his assistants to operate, insisting on doing all procedures himself, hence the impetus for good retraction of the tissues! To avoid damaging the liver, a swab or pack is often placed between the blade of the retractor and the surface of the liver. The exact year that the retractor was introduced is uncertain but it is pictured in an article Deaver wrote on ovarian cancer in 1928 in the *Journal of the American Medical Association* (Deaver 1928).

John Blair Deaver (1855–1931)

Deaver was born in Lancaster County, Pennsylvania, the son of a country doctor. He graduated from the University of Pennsylvania, America's first medical school, in 1878. After internships at the Germantown Hospital and Philadelphia Children's Hospital, he entered clinical practice but continued to work as an anatomy demonstrator at the University of Pennsylvania, later becoming Assistant Professor of Applied Anatomy. In 1886, he took up a post at the Lankenau Hospital in Philadelphia (formerly the German Hospital), where he developed a vast surgical practice. According to *The New York Times*, in one year alone he performed 450 appendicectomies. In 1909 he hosted a dinner for 200 of his ex-patients, 160 of whom had had an appendicectomy performed by him.

He was appointed Professor of Surgery at the University of Pennsylvania Medical School in 1911. His dedication to surgery was outstanding. Although he joined his wife and four children for summer holidays in Maine, he would often return to Philadelphia after less than a week, maintaining that his presence was urgently needed at the hospital! The University twice extended the age limit for compulsory retirement in order to retain his services. Deaver was a founder member of the American College of Surgeons and its president between 1921 and 1922.

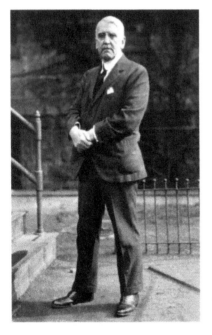

John Blair Deaver. (Courtesy of the University of
Pennsylvania School of Medicine)

He was described as an aggressive and radical surgeon and was an early advocate
of urgent appendicectomy for acute appendicitis. "Cut well, get well, stay well,"

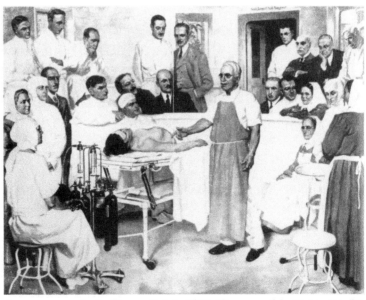

Dr Deaver about to operate in the Deaver clinic in 1928. (Courtesy of the University of Pennsylvania
School of Medicine)

The New York Times. Monday February 1, 1909

was one of his many aphorisms. He had a sharp wit: on one occasion responding to the comment that a surgeon should possess the "heart of a lion, the eye of an eagle, and the hand of a woman" he added "and the constitution of a mule." Deaver wrote widely on many surgical topics; his writings on abdominal surgery included a classic paper on lumbar versus iliac colostomy, and books on appendicitis (1896) and surgical anatomy (1899), both of which ran to several editions.

References

Deaver JB. Papillary cyst carcinoma of the ovary. *JAMA* 1928;**91**:1008–12.

Further reading

Anon. An Appendixless Dinner. 160 Will Dine the Man Who Cut Out Their Appendices. *The New York Times*. Monday February 1, 1909.

Corman ML. John Blair Deaver 1855–1931. *Dis Colon Rectum* 1987;**30**:66–71.

Deaver JB. Lumbar versus iliac colotomy. *Phila Co Med Soc* 1881;**12**:97–106.

Powell JL. John Blair Deaver, MD (1855–1931). *J Pelvic Surg* 2001;7:56–7.

D | Desjardins gallstone forceps

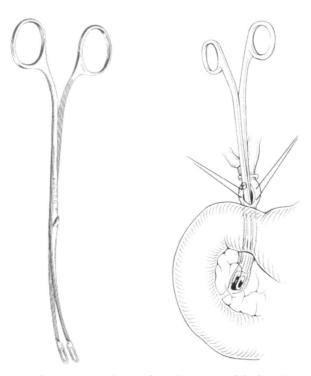

Desjardins gallstone forceps for retrieving gallstones from the common bile duct. (From Carter DC. Cholecystectomy, cholecystostomy and exploration of the common bile duct. In: Carter DC et al, eds. *Rob & Smith's Operative Surgery. Hepatobiliary and Pancreatic Surgery.* 5th edition. Chapman & Hall Medical, London, 1996, p.349. With permission of Hodder Education).

Desjardins gallstone forceps are used to retrieve gallstones during open exploration of the common bile duct, often in conjunction with a biliary balloon catheter. The forceps were designed by Abel Desjardins, not Desjardin as sometimes stated.

Abel Desjardins (1871–1955)

Desjardins trained under Louis-Félix Terrier (1837–1908) at the Pitié-Salpêtrière Hospital in Paris. He became Professor of Surgery in Paris, specialising in hepatobiliary and pancreatic surgery. During his career he worked at both the Pitié Salpêtrière and the Henri de Rothschild Hospitals. Later in his career, he was President of the Society of Surgeons of Paris.

In addition to his gallstone forceps, Desjardins' name is also associated with numerous other biliary tract instruments including a gallstone scoop, bile duct probe and liver retractor. He developed one of the first operative approaches to pancreaticoduodenectomy, albeit in cadavers. The procedure involved a resection of the head of the pancreas and duodenum with gastric, biliary and pancreatic drainage.

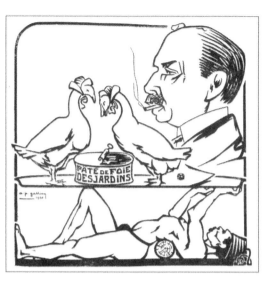

A sketch of Abel Desjardins from the satirical Parisian journal Le Rictus in 1920 © Bibliothèque Interuniversitaire de Médecine de Paris. One goose asks another: "Do you think that that [the pâté de foie Desjardins] is as good as ours?"

Although he never undertook the operation in a patient, he was the first to describe the technique of invaginating the pancreatic stump into the end of a jejunal limb.

Abel Desjardins lived with his family in the fashionable Passy district of Paris, where he was acquainted with Parisian intellectuals and artists, including the writer Marcel Proust (a childhood friend) and the composer Maurice Ravel. Desjardins married Marie Escudier, a well connected society woman who had previously been the wife of a wealthy Parisian industrialist and art patron. A painting of her by the artist Odilon Redon hangs in the Metropolitan Museum of Art in New York under the name of Madame Arthur Fontaine. As well as his cultural and intellectual pursuits, Desjardins was a fierce opponent of animal experiments, maintaining that surgical research achieved nothing from them.

References

Carter DC. Cholecystectomy, cholecystostomy and exploration of the common bile duct. In: Carter DC *et al*, eds. *Rob & Smith's Operative Surgery. Hepatobiliary and Pancreatic Surgery*. 5th edition. Chapman & Hall Medical, London, 1996, p.349.

Further reading

Bibliothèque Interuniversitaire de Médecine de Paris (http://www.bium.univ-paris5.fr/histmed/hm_img.htm) for a catalogue of Desjardin's instruments. Last accessed February 2009.

Desjardins A. Technique de la pancréatectomie. *Rev Chir* 1907;**35**:945–73.

Schnelldorfer T, Adams DB, Warshaw AL, Lillemoe KD, Sarr MG. Forgotten pioneers of pancreatic surgery: beyond the favorite few. *Ann Surg* 2008;**247**:191–202.

D Space of Disse

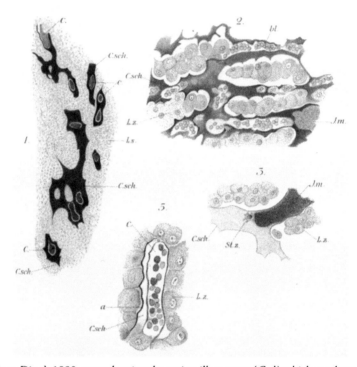

Drawings from Disse's 1890 paper showing the pericapillary space (*Csch*) which was later named the space of Disse. (From Disse J. Ueber die Lymphbahnen der Säugethierleber. *Archiv fur mikroskopische Anatomie*. 1890;36:203–24, plate 10. Courtesy of Niedersächsische Staats-und Universitätsbibliothek, Göttingen).

The space of Disse is the perisinusoidal space in the liver between the fenestrated sinusoidal endothelium and the hepatocyte plates. The sinusoidal endothelium lacks a basal lamina. The space is normally up to 0.5 mm wide and contains interstitial fluid, fibroblasts, collagen fibrils, stellate cells (the fat storing cells of Ito), and unmyelinated nerve terminals.

Disse's 1890 publication on the liver stemmed from research he had been doing in lizards and snakes (Disse 1890). Subcutaneous injection of India ink in these animals produced discolouration of the liver due to the accumulation of ink particles in the spaces between the sinusoids and the hepatocytes. Further injection studies in cats and dogs revealed that these spaces communicated with periportal lymphatics.

Joseph Hugo Vincent Disse (1852–1912)

Disse was a German anatomist and histologist. He obtained his doctorate in medicine in 1875 from the University of Erlangen and, after postgraduate study in anatomy

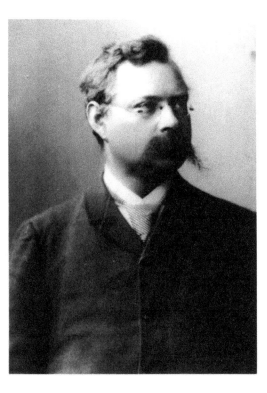

Joseph Hugo Vincent Disse. (Courtesy of
Universitätsarchiv in Halle, Germany)

at Strasbourg University he took up a post as Professor of Anatomy at the University
of Tokyo, remaining there between 1880 and 1888. Upon his return to Germany he
worked as a junior faculty member at the Anatomical Institute at the University of
Göttingen. It was from here that he published his paper on 'The Lymphatic Tracts of
the Mammalian Liver'. In 1895 he moved to the University of Marburg, where he
became Professor of Anatomy and Director of the university's anatomical institute.
He died in 1912 from tuberculosis.

Disse specialised in gross and comparative anatomy, embryology and histology.
His published works included studies on the paranasal sinuses, the evolution of the
olfactory nerve, and the microanatomy of the gastric mucosa, kidneys and teeth.

Reference

Disse J. Ueber die Lymphbahnen der Säugethierleber. *Archiv fur mikroskopische Anatomie*.
1890;**36**:203–24.

Further reading

Schmid R. Who was Disse? *Hepatology* 1991;**14**:1283–5.

DuVal procedure for chronic pancreatitis

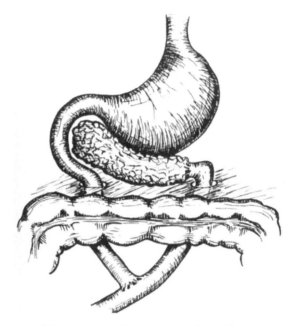

Schematic representation of the anatomy at the conclusion of DuVal's operation. (From DuVal MK. Caudal pancreatico-jejunostomy for chronic relapsing pancreatitis. *Ann Surg* 1954;140:775–85, Fig. 1, p.777. © Lippincott Williams & Wilkins)

DuVal's procedure for the surgical treatment of chronic pancreatitis involves resection of the tail of the pancreas, splenectomy and retrograde drainage of the main pancreatic duct into a defunctioned Roux-en-Y limb of jejunum. The pancreaticojejunostomy is fashioned in two layers: an inner duct-to-duct mucosal anastomosis using fine catgut sutures and an outer layer of interrupted silk sutures.

The concept behind the operation was that proximal pancreatic duct obstruction causes chronic pancreatitis and that the obstructed duct can be decompressed in such cases via the tail of the gland. In his 1954 paper he reported two patients who underwent this procedure; they were both only followed up for a few weeks but measures of pancreatic exocrine function did seem to improve (DuVal 1954). A further report in 1961 documented results in 28 patients followed for periods of up to 8 years. Pain relief was achieved in two-thirds of the patients (DuVal 1961).

DuVal's procedure met with less success in the hands of others, probably because it failed to address the common problem of multiple strictures of the proximal pancreatic duct in chronic pancreatitis. It was largely abandoned in favour of Puestow's procedure (1958) (see Puestow procedure, p. 158) and other more comprehensive drainage operations.

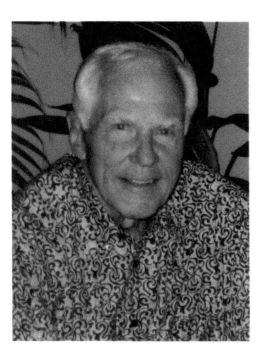

Merlin DuVal Jr pictured in 2006. (Courtesy of Dartmouth Medical School Publications)

Merlin K. DuVal Jr (1922–)

Merlin K. DuVal Jr graduated from Dartmouth College and Medical School in 1944 and obtained his MD from Cornell University in 1946. After service in the Navy, he completed his surgical residency with Dr Allen O. Whipple (1881–1963) in New York, who stimulated his interest in pancreatic surgery. DuVal joined the surgery faculty of the State University of New York and while working in Brooklyn he implemented his innovative surgical procedure to treat chronic pancreatitis. In 1957 he moved to the University of Oklahoma School of Medicine, where he became particularly interested in medical education. DuVal gave up his surgical practice in the early 1960s in order to establish Arizona's first medical school in Tucson. He later served as US Assistant Secretary of Health and was active in health care politics before retiring in 1990.

References

DuVal MK. Caudal pancreatico-jejunostomy for chronic relapsing pancreatitis. *Ann Surg* 1954;**140**:775–85.

DuVal MK Jr, Enquist IF. The surgical treatment of chronic pancreatitis by pancreaticojejunostomy: an 8-year reappraisal. *Surgery* 1961;**50**:965–9.

DuVal procedure for chronic pancreatitis

Further reading

Carter LS. Merlin DuVal, M.D. '44: On the ball. *Dartmouth Medicine.* Spring 2006, pp54–7. http://dartmed.dartmouth.edu/spring06/html/alumni_album.php (Last accessed 16/1/09).

Wani NA, Parray FQ, Wani MA. Is any surgical procedure ideal for chronic pancreatitis? *Int J Surg* 2007;**5**:45–56.

Frey procedure for chronic pancreatitis

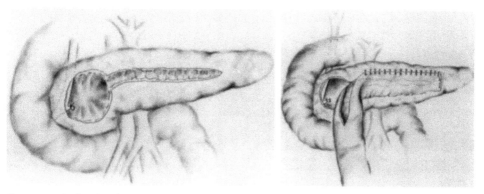

Coring out the head and uncinate process and filleting the main pancreatic duct, which is drained into a jejunal Roux loop. (From Frey CF, Smith GJ. Description and rationale of a new operation for chronic pancreatitis. *Pancreas* 1987;**2**:701–7, Fig. 1 p.702 and Fig. 2 p.703. © Lippincott, Williams & Wilkins)

The ideal operation for chronic pancreatitis should provide long-term pain relief, be as simple and safe as possible, and preserve residual endocrine and exocrine pancreatic function. On this basis, Frey devised a new operative procedure for chronic pancreatitis and reported the outcome in six patients in 1987. Pre-existing procedures all had major limitations:

1. Total pancreatectomy was radical, potentially hazardous, and resulted in disabling pancreatic insufficiency;
2. Pancreaticoduodenectomy provided good pain relief but produced metabolic disturbances and carried a risk of operative mortality;
3. A distal pancreatectomy was useful but mostly in patients with disease limited to the body or tail of the gland;
4. Longitudinal pancreaticojejunostomy (Partington–Rochelle modification), although often successful, was associated with recurrent pain in up to one-third of patients because of incomplete decompression of the pancreatic ductal system within the head of the pancreas.

Local resection of the pancreatic head combined with longitudinal pancreatico-jejunostomy (the Frey procedure) removes diseased tissue within the head of the pancreas, and decompresses the entire pancreatic duct system. It preserves pancreatic parenchyma and does not entail duodenal or bile duct surgery or pancreatic transection with their attendant risks.

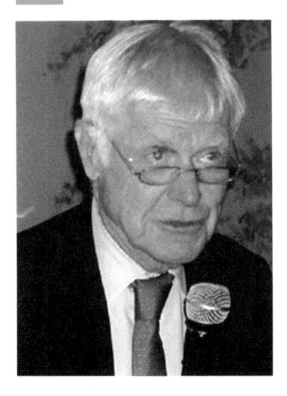

Charles F. Frey. (Courtesy of the Pancreas Club, Inc. USA)

Charles Frederick Frey (1929–)

Born in New York he obtained his MD from Cornell University in 1955. His training in general surgery was punctuated by a two-year stint in the United States Air Force. He became Professor of Surgery at the University of Michigan, where he worked with Charles Gardner Child (1908–1991). It was here that he witnessed the results of Child's 95% distal pancreatectomy and observed that whilst it was effective at relieving pain, a high proportion of patients developed pancreatic insufficiency.

Frey moved to the University of California in 1976, where he was Vice Chair of Surgery and it was here that he conceived of the Frey procedure for chronic pancreatitis (a procedure he modestly refers to as 'local resection of the head of the pancreas combined with longitudinal pancreaticojejunostomy'). He retired in 1997, having achieved an international reputation in pancreatic surgery. He chaired the Pancreas Club in the United States from 1975 to 1995.

References

Frey CF, Smith GJ. Description and rationale of a new operation for chronic pancreatitis. *Pancreas* 1987;**2**:701–7.

Further reading

Frey CF, Reber HA. Local resection of the head of the pancreas with pancreaticojejunostomy. *J Gastrointest Surg* 2005;**9**:863–8.

Frey CF, Schiller W. Introduction to the history of the Pancreas Club, Inc. *J Gastrointest Surg* 2004;8(Suppl 2):S1.

Ho HS, Frey CF. The Frey procedure: local resection of pancreatic head combined with lateral pancreaticojejunostomy. *Arch Surg* 2001;**136**:1353–8.

Partington PF, Rochelle RL. Modified Puestow procedure for retrograde drainage of the pancreatic duct. *Ann Surg* 1969:**152**:1037–43.

Peskin GW. The pancreas. A symposium in honor of Charles Frederick Frey, MD. *Arch Surg* 1998;**133**:223–5.

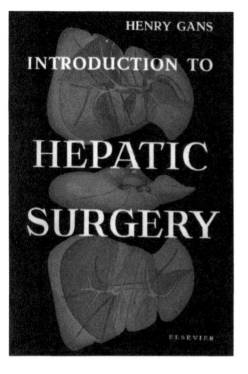

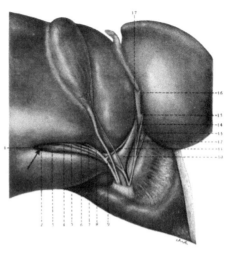

The fissure of Gans highlighted by the arrow in this inferior view of the liver (label 2. incisura dextra in the original figure). (From Gans H. Introduction to Hepatic Surgery. Elsevier, Amsterdam, 1955. Fig. 25, p.52. © Elsevier 1955)

Gans studied the anatomy of the liver from corrosion casts and in 1955 published a book entitled *Introduction to Hepatic Surgery*, summarising anatomical approaches to liver resections. In this he described the 'incisura dextra', which has since become known as the fissure of Gans (Gans 1955). This is a groove on the inferior surface of the liver near the bed of the gall bladder and often marks the rather variable division of the right pedicle of Glisson's sheath and portal triad, where it gives off the inferior segment VI division of the posterolateral sectoral branch. In one study, the fissure was found in 73% of livers (Reynaud et al 1991). This can be a useful landmark for isolating the posterolateral sectoral triad or its segment VI subdivision during hepatic resections.

Henry Gans (1925–)

Gans was born in Zevenaar in the Netherlands. As a schoolboy in 1942 in Nazi-occupied Holland, he recalls the persecution of Jews and his fortunate protection by a Dutch farmer. During junior surgical training, he decided to study the anatomy of the liver after discovering that his mother had inoperable liver cancer. Working in Nijmegen in the Netherlands, he recounts that "In not much more than a year, we injected and studied almost a hundred livers, evaluated the surgical approaches to the lobar and segmental structures, oversaw the photography and drawing of more than 10 dozen original illustrations, negotiated with Elsevier for the publication of a

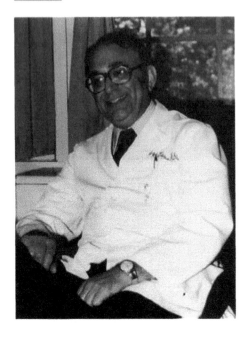

Henry Gans. (Picture taken in the late 1970s kindly provided by Dr Gans)

book, and read more than 500 surgical papers before publishing a thesis." His text on liver surgery was published in 1955, whilst he was a surgical resident in Cincinnati, Ohio. This was two years before Couinaud's book on the anatomy of the liver. Not only did Gans' text provide a rational anatomical basis for liver resection but he also made the clinically important observation that hepatic metastases received their blood supply from the hepatic artery.

Gans's later research focused more on haemostasis and endotoxins; he demonstrated that endotoxaemia was associated with the development of disseminated intravascular coagulation. He maintained his interest in liver surgery and, in 1969, together with colleagues at New York Hospital Cornell Medical Center, he performed two reduced-sized liver transplants; in both cases the left lobe of the donor liver was resected ex-vivo to produce a better donor-recipient size match. This was some 14 years before Bismuth and Houssin performed a reduced-size liver transplant in a child using the left lobe from an adult donor liver (Bismuth and Houssin 1984).

Gans retired from his post as Professor of Surgery, Pathology and Biochemistry at the University of Illinois College of Medicine in 1984.

References

Bismuth H, Houssin D. Reduced-sized orthotopic liver graft in hepatic transplantation in children. *Surgery* 1984;**95**:367–70.

Gans H. *Introduction to Hepatic Surgery*. Elsevier, Amsterdam, 1955.

Reynaud BH, Coucoravas GO, Giuly JA. Basis to improve several hepatectomy techniques involving the surgical anatomy of incisura dextra of Gans. *Surg Gynecol Obstet* 1991;**172**:490–2.

Further reading

Gans H. Circumstance and serendipity. *Surgery* 2001;**130**:82–4.

Gans H. Development of modern liver surgery. *Lancet* 2002;**360**:805.

Gans H. A thank you to an old Dutch farmer. *Lancet* 2004;**364**:2095–6.

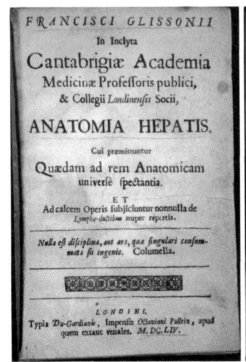
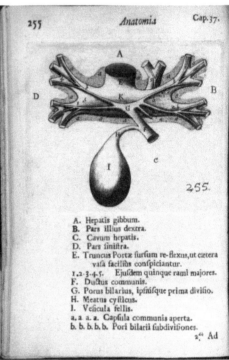

Title page and illustration of the porta hepatis (p.255, cap 37) from Francis Glisson's *Anatomia Hepatis. Cui praemittuntur Quaedam ad rem Anatomicam universe spectantia. Et Ad calcem Operis subjiciuntur nonnulla de Lymphae-ductibus nuper repertis.* Typis Du-Gardianis, Impensis Octaviani Pullein, Londini, 1654 [The Anatomy of the Liver, prefaced by some matters of general anatomical importance. And to this work is added something concerning the lymph ducts only recently discovered]. (Reproduced with permission of Leeds University Library, UK)

Glisson's *Anatomia Hepatis* published in 1654 provided a detailed account of the normal and morbid anatomy of the liver (Glisson 1654). In it, he described the connective tissue that surrounds the portal vein, hepatic artery and hepatic ducts at the porta hepatis, and the extension of this sheath into the liver parenchyma. This is continuous with the external covering of the liver and is known as Glisson's capsule. *Anatomia Hepatis* was the first book printed in England which gave a detailed account of a single organ based on original research.

Glisson's sheath or capsule had previously been described by the anatomist Johannes Walaeus (alt. Valoeus) of Brussels in 1640 but Glisson is rightly credited with the detailed description of the extension of the capsule at the hilum into the liver parenchyma around the portal triads.

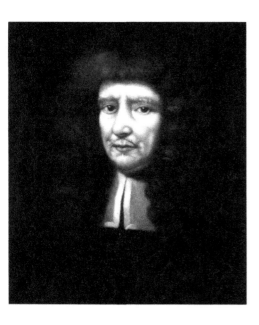

Portrait of Francis Glisson attributed to
William Faithorne and painted before 1672.
(Courtesy of the Heritage Centre, Royal
College of Physicians, London)

Francis Glisson (1598–1677)

Francis Glisson was an important figure in seventeenth century medicine. He was born in Dorset (in 1598 or 1599 according to Walker) and educated at Caius College, Cambridge, where he lectured in Greek. He did not begin his medical studies until he was 30 years old and obtained his medical degree from Cambridge in 1634. William Harvey, a previous student from the same Cambridge College, had recently published his *Exercitatio Anatomica de Motu Cordis et Sanguinis in Animalibus* (1628) and declared that wise men must learn anatomy, not from the wisdom of philosophers but from nature itself.

In 1635, Glisson was elected Fellow of the College of Physicians, where he lectured on anatomy and medicine. In 1636, he was appointed Regius Professor of Physics at Cambridge, a post he occupied until his death. However, he lived most of his life in London, surviving both the Great Plague in 1665 and the Great Fire in 1666. Glisson eventually became president of the College of Physicians in London*(1667–1669) and was one of the first Fellows of the Royal Society.

Glisson described other aspects of hepatobiliary anatomy including the vasculature of the liver (derived from injection casts). In the absence of any microscopy he deduced that portal blood traversed the 'capillaries' in the liver to reach the vena cava. He also included an account of the lymphatics of the liver as communicated to him by George Jolyffe and he noted the existence of a sphincter around the termination of the common bile duct (later referred to as the sphincter of Oddi).

73

His other published works included a treatise on infantile rickets (1650), a philosophical treatise on the nature of life (1672), and a book on the stomach and intestines (1677). He was married but had no children. Glisson was buried at St Bride's church in London.

*The College was founded in 1518 and acquired its Royal prefix in 1674.

References

Glisson F. *Anatomia Hepatis*. Du-Gardianis, Impensis Octaviani Pullein, Londini, 1654.

Further reading

Dunn PM. Francis Glisson (1597–1677) and the 'discovery' of rickets. *Arch Dis Child Fetal Neonatal Ed* 1998;**78**:F154–F155.

Jones AR. Francis Glisson. *J Bone Joint Surg (Br)* 1950:**32-B**:425–8.

Walker RM. Francis Glisson and his capsule. *Ann R Coll Surg Engl* 1966;**38**:71–91.

Wood M. Eponyms in biliary tract surgery. *Am J Surg* 1979;**138**:746–54.

Grey Turner's sign in acute pancreatitis

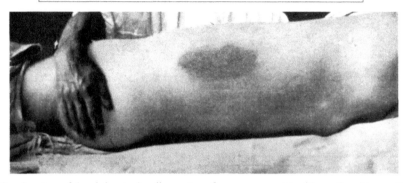

Within the image:

THE BRITISH JOURNAL OF SURGERY

LOCAL DISCOLORATION OF THE ABDOMINAL WALL AS A SIGN OF ACUTE PANCREATITIS.

By G. GREY TURNER, Newcastle-on-Tyne.

Local discoloration of the abdominal wall as a sign of acute pancreatitis. (From Grey Turner G. Local discoloration of the abdominal wall as a sign of acute pancreatitis. *Br J Surg* 1919;27:394–5. © British Journal of Surgery Society Ltd. Reproduced with permission of John Wiley & Sons Ltd)

Grey Turner's description of discolouration of the abdominal wall in acute pancreatitis was published in 1919. He described two patients with fatal necrotising pancreatitis. The first had an area of bluish discolouration in about a 6 in (15 cm) diameter around the umbilicus and the second (pictured above) had a greenish discolouration in the loins. He attributed the discolouration to retroperitoneal inflammation spreading along the falciform ligament or directly to the flanks.

George Grey Turner (1877–1951)

Born in North Shields, North East England, George Grey Turner was the second of five sons of James Grey Turner, a bank clerk, and his wife, Evelyn. He gained a scholarship to Newcastle Upon Tyne Medical School (then part of Durham University) and graduated in 1898. After resident surgical posts in Newcastle, he undertook postgraduate studies at King's College Hospital, London and in Vienna before returning to Newcastle in 1906, where he was appointed to the staff of the Royal Victoria Infirmary. He was greatly influenced by the Professor of Surgery, Rutherford Morison (1853–1939)(see Morison's pouch, p. 136).

75

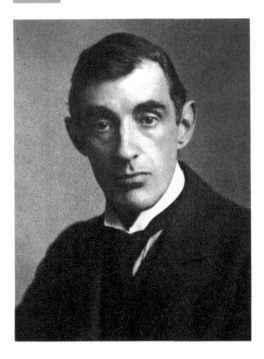

George Grey Turner (circa 1920) from the Council album. (Reproduced by kind permission of the President and Council of the Royal College of Surgeons of England)

As a young surgeon Grey Turner operated not only at the Infirmary but in nursing homes and patients' cottages, when he would perform operations on the kitchen table with a country doctor providing the anaesthetic. By the outbreak of war in 1914, Grey Turner was Senior Surgeon and he served with the Royal Army Medical Corps in the Middle East, rising to the rank of colonel. He made one of the earliest attempts to remove a bullet from a soldier's heart; the bullet was never removed, but the patient survived and Grey Turner subsequently became a specialist in chest surgery to the Northern Command in England. After the war he returned to his post at the Royal Victoria Infirmary in Newcastle, becoming Professor of Surgery at Durham University in 1927.

When the British Postgraduate Medical School was opened in Hammersmith, London, in 1935 Grey Turner was appointed as the Director of Surgery and remained there until 1946, when he was succeeded by Ian Aird (1905–1962).

Grey Turner was a true general surgeon but his special interests included cancer (which he deemed would not be overcome by surgery but by "something we will inject") and congenital malformations of the bladder. He was one of the first to succeed in urinary diversion into the colon. He was well known for experience with block dissection of the neck, perineal excision of the rectum, colectomy, oesophageal surgery and cleft palate repair.

G

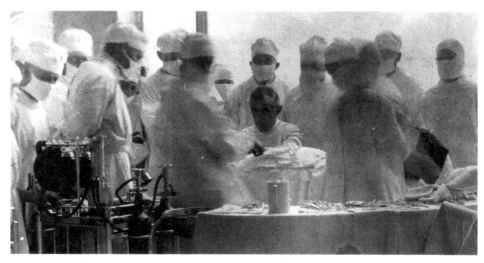

Professor Grey Turner in the operating theatre circa 1936. (By kind permission of the Royal Postgraduate Medical School archives and the Archives and Corporate Records Unit, Imperial College London)

Turner was a short man who dressed almost invariably in a black coat and striped trousers and, on the back of his large head, he wore an old bowler hat which he also used to keep his tea warm! He wore heavy boots with thick soles and, in winter, knitted mittens. His appearance amused his friends but he never took offence. He was courteous and kind and much respected by colleagues and patients alike. In 1908 he married Alice (Elsie) Grey, with whom he had four children.

He received many honours, serving on the Council of the Royal College of Surgeons of England between 1926 and 1950, becoming Vice-president in 1937, and holding office at the Royal Society of Medicine and International Society of Surgery. He was very knowledgeable about John Hunter and his legacy and, in addition to a Hunterian professorship in 1928, he was a Hunterian orator (in 1945) and elected Trustee of the Hunterian Collection (in 1951). He was instrumental in reorganising the collection after much of it was destroyed by bombing during World War II.

Grey Turner travelled widely and visited North and South America, Australia, Africa, and Europe; he was a prolific writer and published several hundred papers. He gave the Murphy oration in Philadelphia in 1930 and was awarded the Bigelow Medal in Boston in 1931. He was an honorary fellow of the American College of Surgeons and the Royal Australasian College of Surgeons, received honorary degrees from Glasgow and Durham together with an honorary fellowship from the Royal College of Surgeons of Edinburgh, and was a Freeman of the City of London.

Grey Turner's sign in acute pancreatitis

References

Grey Turner G. Local discoloration of the abdominal wall as a sign of acute pancreatitis. *Br J Surg* 1919;**27**:394–5.

Further reading

In memoriam. George Grey Turner. *Br J Surg* 1951;**39**:193–4.

Obituary. G Grey Turner, MS, LLD (Hon), DCh (Hon), FRCS. *Br Med J* 1951;**ii**:550–3.

Wakeley C, Booth CC. George Grey Turner. *Oxford Dictionary of National Biography* 2004. http://www.oxforddnb.com/index/101036585/ (Last accessed October 2008).

White H. An outstanding ISS/SIC Surgeon: George Grey Turner. *World J Surg* 2003;**27**:511–13.

H Hartmann's pouch

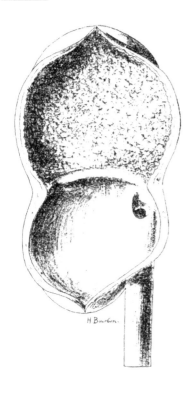

H Bourbon.

Hartmann's pouch. (From Hartmann H. Quelques points l'anatomie et de la chirurgie des voies biliaires. *Bull Soc Anat Paris* 1891;5:480–500. Fig. 4, p.491. © Société Anatomique de Paris)

In 1891, Hartmann* described his now famous gall bladder pouch in the region of the gall bladder that Paul Broca had previously called the "gall bladder basin". Hartmann noted that the gall bladder typically had a dilated ampullary region proximal to the origin of the cystic duct. This ampulla was separated from the body of the gall bladder by an external groove and an internal mucosal fold. Hartmann's pouch arises from distortion and distension of the ampulla caused by an impacted gallstone; this produces a cul-de-sac below the origin of the cystic duct. Hartmann found this to have been present in five of 14 gall bladders operated on for stone disease.

*Hartmann's solution is named after Alexis Hartmann (1898–1964), an American paediatrician who introduced this intravenous fluid (also known as lactated Ringer's solution) in the 1930s.

Henri Albert Hartmann (1860–1952)

Henri Albert Charles Antoine Hartmann was born in Paris, where he lived throughout his life. His family had a strong work ethic. He graduated from the University of Paris in 1881, became an anatomy prosector in 1886, a surgeon in 1892, and a full professor of surgery in 1909. Among his mentors was the renowned surgeon,

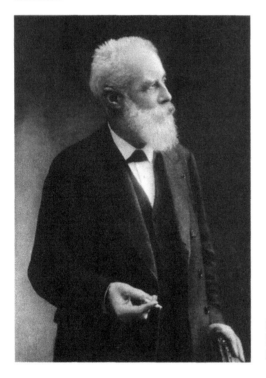

Henri Albert Hartmann. (Courtesy of the Bibliotheque de l'Academie Nationale de Médecine, Paris)

Louis-Félix Terrier (1837–1908), from whom he learned the importance of asepsis and a commitment to hard work, integrity and respect for the patient. Hartmann progressed to become Chief of Surgery at the Hôtel-Dieu Hospital on the banks of the river Seine in 1914. Here he performed more than 1000 operations a year for over 20 years. He was an extremely eminent French surgeon and through his work and visits abroad he was awarded many honours and distinctions. He received an honorary fellowship of the Royal College of Surgeons of England in 1913 and of the American Surgical Association and the French Legion of Honour. He became President of the French Academy of Medicine in 1936.

Hartmann was well read and had a large personal library of surgical literature. He kept meticulous surgical notes and carefully retained operative specimens in a small museum adjacent to his library. He wrote extensively on many topics including the surgical anatomy of the rectum and biliary tract, gynaecology, and cancer of the stomach and rectum. His operation for cancer of the rectosigmoid region first described in 1921 is still widely known as Hartmann's procedure (Ronel and Hardy 2002). His operative techniques were always underpinned by a sound knowledge of anatomy and pathology.

Hartmann respected progress and was not afraid to change his opinion about the best approach to a surgical problem. However, he could be sarcastic and humiliating toward his students and was prone to outbursts of temper. "He disliked laziness,

80

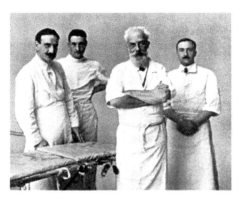

Henri Hartmann at Hôtel Dieu, Paris, July 1920 with his assistants. (From Br J Surg 1920;8:223. By permission of John Wiley & Sons Ltd)

boastfulness, and idleness, and if in the course of his gallops across the courtyards of l'Hôtel-Dieu or when flying up a flight of stairs he ran into a smoker, gossips, or young lovers he would let explode the most formidable expletives". He operated in silence and only conveyed tension during an operation by bumping into his assistants. He rarely took vacations. Hartmann was married but had no children. On 1 January 1952, at the age of 91, he slipped and fell down stairs, dying the next day. He is buried in the Père-Lachaise cemetery in Paris.

References

Hartmann H. Quelques points l'anatomie et de la chirurgie des voies biliaires. *Bull Soc Anat Paris* 1891;**5**:480–500.

Ronel DN, Hardy MA. Henri Albert Hartmann: labor and discipline. *Current Surgery* 2002;**59**: 59–64.

Further reading

Anon. A visit to the clinic of Professor Henri Hartmann, at the Hôtel Dieu, Paris, July 1920. *Br J Surg* 1920;**8**:223–5.

Monod MR. Notice nécrologique sur le professeur Henri Hartmann. *Bull Acad Nat Med Paris* 1952;**136**:201–4.

Moulonguet P. Henri Hartmann (1860–1952). *J Chirurgie* 1952;**68**:169–76.

Patel J. Potraits de Chirurgiens de l'Hôtel-Dieu. *Presse Méd* 1959;**60**:2317–20.

H Heister's spiral 'valve'

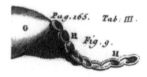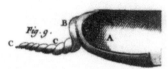

Heister's drawing of the cystic duct and spiral valve from the 1748 edition of his *Compendium Anatomicum* (Fig. 9, Volume 2, p.165)

In 1717, Lorenz Heister published his *Compendium of Anatomy*, in which he described a spiral "valve" in the cystic duct. Whilst no longer regarded as a valve, the function of these spiral mucosal folds remains obscure. Typically, the mucous membrane of the cystic duct has between two and ten crescentic folds projecting into its lumen along the length of the duct, being larger and more concentrated in its proximal portion. Similar folds are an inconstant finding in the terminal segment of the gall bladder neck. The folds are arranged more or less spirally in the majority of cystic ducts, usually run in a clockwise direction down the duct and interdigitate with folds on the opposite wall. Most of the folds extend 50–75% of the way around the duct lumen but some make one or even two complete circuits. Occasionally, the folds are totally absent. At the other extreme, as many as 22 folds have been recorded in healthy biliary tracts. Dasgupta and Stringer (2005) suggested that the spiral folds may help to preserve the patency and calibre of the cystic duct rather than regulate the flow of bile, i.e. they may be a structural device rather than acting as a valvular mechanism.

Lorenz Heister (1683–1758)

Heister was born in Frankfurt am Main, Germany, where he attended the Latin school and excelled in the arts, music, languages and painting. He was so gifted that his father, a merchant, decided to invest in a university education for his son. In 1702, Heister began his medical studies at the University of Giessen. In 1706, he moved to the Netherlands to study botany in Leiden and anatomy in Amsterdam with Frederick Ruysch (1638–1731). He commented: "During which time I was also employed in frequent dissections, and in trying chirurgical operations upon dead subjects". He obtained his doctorate in medicine in 1708 from the University of Harderwijk (Netherlands), submitting a thesis on the choroid of the eye. A year later he joined the Dutch Army as a field surgeon and gained intensive experience in several military campaigns. In 1711 he was appointed Professor of Surgery and Anatomy at the University of Altdorf near Nuremberg in Germany. Prior to taking up this position he visited several medical centres in England. In 1719 he was appointed

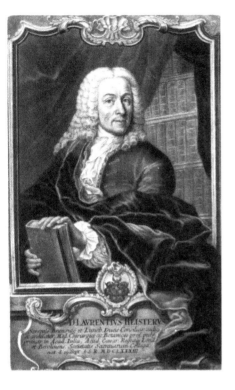

Lorenz Heister. (From an engraving by M.W. Froling)

to the Chair of Anatomy and Surgery at the University of Helmstädt, where he later also became Professor of Botany. He was elected to the Royal Society of London in 1730.

Heister published a major influential text, *Chirurgie* [Surgery] in 1718 and is regarded by many as the founder of scientific surgery in Germany. He condemned texts of surgery written by those who had studied little anatomy or who had had little practical experience. In 1717 he published his *Compendium of Anatomy*, a companion text to his Surgery, which was written in Latin but subsequently translated into many languages and revised in some 25 editions.

His other works included treatises on ophthalmology and botany. In 1753, he published the first detailed postmortem description of perforated appendicitis. He is credited with the introduction of the spinal brace and coining the term 'tracheotomy'.

Heister had a famous botanical garden in Helmstädt and his name is given to the plant genus *Heisteria*. He was married with one son. He is buried in St Stephan's cemetery in Helmstädt, Germany.

Heister's spiral 'valve'

References

Dasgupta D, Stringer MD. Cystic duct and Heister's "valves". *Clin Anat* 2005;**18**:81–7.

Heister L. *Compendium Anatomicum Totam Rem Anatomicam*. Volume 2, GC Weber, Nürnberg, 1748, p. 165.

Further reading

Bird NC, Ooi RC, Luo XY, Chin SB, Johnson AG. Investigation of the functional three-dimensional anatomy of the human cystic duct: A single helix? *Clin Anat* 2006;**19**:528–34.

Editorial. Lorenz Heister (1683–1758) Eighteenth century surgeon. *JAMA* 1967;**202**:136–7.

Heister L. *Medical, Chirurgical and Anatomical Cases and Observations* (German). J C Koppe, Rostock, Germany, 1753.

Mentzer SH. The valves of Heister. *Arch Surg* 1926;**13**:511–22.

Wood M. Eponyms in biliary tract surgery. *Am J Surg* 1979;**138**:746–54.

Zimmerman LM, Veith I. *Great Ideas in the History of Surgery*. Lorenz Heister (1683–1758). Norman Publishing, CA, 1993, pp313–23.

H | Canals of Hering

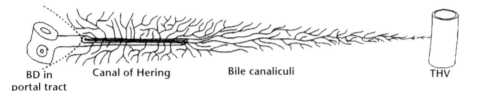

BD in portal tract   Canal of Hering   Bile canaliculi   THV

A schematic of the canal of Hering forming a trough-like structure within the liver lobule and draining bile from bile canaliculi into a bile ductule and terminal bile duct. BD, bile duct; THV, terminal hepatic venule. (From Saxena R, Theise ND, Crawford JM. Microanatomy of the human liver – exploring the hidden interfaces. Hepatology 1999;30:1339–46. Fig. 3b, p.1344. ©1999 John Wiley & Sons. Reprinted with permission of John Wiley & Sons, Inc)

The canals of Hering found within liver lobules are lined by both cholangiocytes and hepatocytes, and convey bile from bile canaliculi to bile ductules, which drain into the terminal bile ducts within portal tracts. Multiple bile canaliculi drain into a single canal. In recent years, it has been shown that the canals of Hering have a trough-like structure. They are also a site where hepatic stem cells are found.

The canals of Hering are difficult to see by light microscopy but Hering described them in various animals in 1866. However, his studies do not mention the human liver. Hering's discovery was greatly overshadowed by his other contributions to physiology and medicine.

Karl Ewald Konstantin Hering (1834–1918)

Ewald Hering was a German physiologist who achieved fame principally through his studies on visual perception, most notably colour vision. His visual theories have since been revised but his other anatomical and physiological discoveries have withstood the test of time.

After graduating from the University of Leipzig in 1860, Hering practised medicine briefly and then returned to physiology. He was appointed to the Chair of Physiology at the Josephs-Akademie in Vienna where, together with Josef Breuer (1842–1925), he discovered the Hering–Breuer reflex, which is activated to prevent overinflation of the lungs.

Hering took up the Chair of Physiology in Prague in 1870 and remained there for 25 years, devoting much of his research to the study of visual perception. He was instrumental in the founding of the German University in Prague. In 1895, he returned to the University of Leipzig.

His son, Heinrich Ewald Hering (1866–1948) became Professor of Physiology at the University of Cologne in Germany and achieved fame through his work on the

85

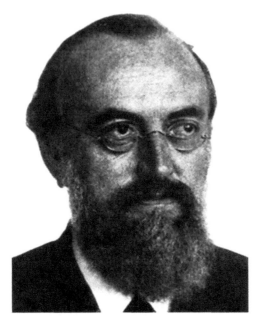

Karl Ewald Konstantin Hering.

carotid sinus baroreceptor reflex (spawning the eponym Hering's nerves – afferent nerve fibres from the carotid sinus within the glossopharyngeal nerve).

References

Saxena R, Theise ND, Crawford JM. Microanatomy of the human liver – exploring the hidden interfaces. *Hepatology* 1999;**30**:1339–46.

Further reading

Hering E. Uber den Bau der Wirbelthierleber. *Archiv fur mikroskopische Anatomie und Entwicklungsmechanik.* 1867;**3**:88–118.

Saxena R, Theise N. Canals of Hering: recent insights and current knowledge. *Semin Liver Dis* 2004;**24**:43–8.

H | Hjortsjö's crook

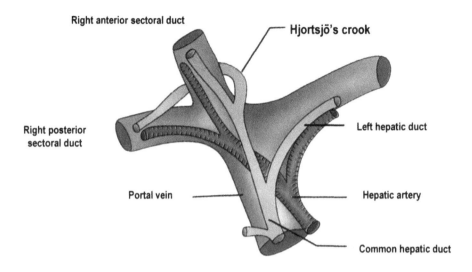

Right anterior sectoral duct

Hjortsjö's crook

Right posterior
sectoral duct

Left hepatic duct

Portal vein

Hepatic artery

Common hepatic duct

Diagrammatic illustration of Hjortsjö's crook

Hjortsjö studied intrahepatic vascular and biliary anatomy from corrosion casts and cholangiograms. In his 1951 paper (Hjortsjö 1951), he described the division of the right hepatic duct into anterior and posterior sectoral ducts (he called the latter the dorsocaudal segment); these followed the corresponding intrahepatic portal vein divisions. In most cases, the posterior sectoral bile duct passed cranial to the anterior sectoral branch of the portal vein and bile duct before running caudally. This created an angled course or hook as the right posterolateral duct curved around the right anteromedial sheath, rendering this duct vulnerable to injury when performing an extended left hepatectomy (left trisectionectomy).

Carl-Herman Hjortsjö (1914–1978)

Carl-Herman Hjortsjö was Director of the Institute of Anatomy in Lund, Sweden. He was an anthropologist and anatomist with a broad range of academic interests.

Hjortsjö studied a diverse range of subjects, which included: human facial expression, about which he wrote a famous book; the skeletal remains of St Bridget, a Swedish fourteenth century saint noted for her morality and mysticism; the burial costume of the seventeenth century Queen Kristina of Sweden; and the development of the mammalian lung.

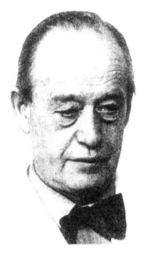 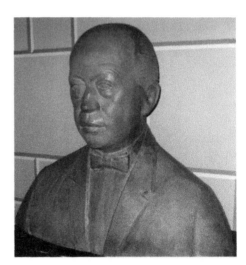

Carl-Herman Hjortsjö. The bust is at the entrance of the former Institute of Anatomy in Lund and was sculpted by Nandor Wagner. (Photograph kindly provided by Gunnar Lundin, Medical Faculty Library, University of Lund)

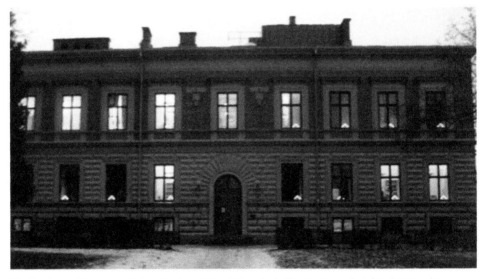

The Institute of Anatomy in Lund, where Hjortsjö worked. The Institute closed in 1980 and is now used as a cultural venue [Kulturanatomen]. Photograph kindly provided by Gunnar Lundin, Medical Faculty Library, University of Lund

References

Hjortsjö CH. The topography of the intrahepatic duct systems. *Acta Anat* 1951;**11**:599–615.

Ito cell

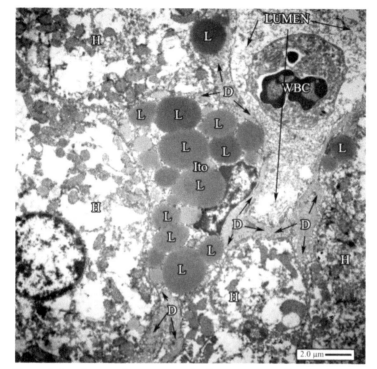

Transmission electron photomicrograph of a primate Ito cell. L, lipid droplet; H, hepatocyte; WBC, white blood cell; D, space of Disse. (Courtesy of Dr Robert Kyle Pope, USA)

Ito cells are hepatic stellate cells found in the perisinusoidal space of Disse in the liver. They typically store vitamin A within lipid droplets in their cytoplasm. Stellate cells are activated by liver injury and are implicated in the pathognesis of hepatic fibrosis. They are also believed to have a role as antigen presenting cells.

Toshio Ito (1904–1991)

Toshio Ito, Professor of Anatomy at Gunma University, Japan, described lipid-containing cells surrounded by reticular fibres in the space of Disse in the human liver lobule. Ito initially called these cells "fat intake cells" but he later concluded that the lipid droplets were derived from glycogen and he changed the name to "fat store cells". The identity of these cells was finally established by Kenjiro Wake, a researcher from Osaka City University Medical School, who determined that the original stellate cells of Kupffer and the lipid-laden cells of Ito were one and the

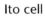

same. The nomenclature of these hepatic stellate cells still remains controversial (Reuben 2002).

Reference

Reuben A. Ito becomes a star. *Hepatology* 2002;**35**:503–4.

K Kasai portoenterostomy

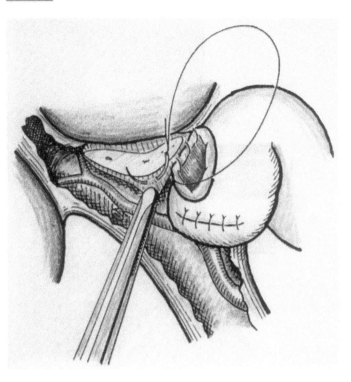

One of Kasai's early
illustrations of his
portoenterostomy
operation for biliary
atresia. (Courtesy of
Professor Ryoji Ohi,
Miyagi Children's
Hospital, Sendai, Japan)

Morio Kasai performed the first hepatic portoenterostomy for so-called 'non-correctable' biliary atresia in 1955. This is the commonest type of biliary atresia – a condition in which infants are born with occluded extrahepatic bile ducts. Unless bile drainage is restored, the child develops progressive liver disease, which is invariably fatal in early childhood. Before the Kasai procedure was developed, only infants with distal bile duct occlusion and proximal extrahepatic duct patency (fewer than 10% of all infants with biliary atresia) had been successfully treated.* Kasai reported his new operative technique in a Japanese journal in 1959 and only later (in 1968) in an English language journal (Kasai 1959, 1968). The hepatic portoenterostomy procedure involves the systematic dissection of the obliterated extrahepatic bile ducts, precise transection of the occluded ductal remnants at the porta hepatis, and anastomosis of a conduit (typically a Roux loop of jejunum) to the raw cut surface of the transected portal plate. The operation is more likely to lead to resolution of jaundice if performed before 3 months of age. In children with biliary atresia, the Kasai portoenterostomy still remains the definitive treatment of choice.

*One of the first such reports of successful surgery was published in 1928 by William E. Ladd (1880–1967), considered by many as the father of paediatric surgery.

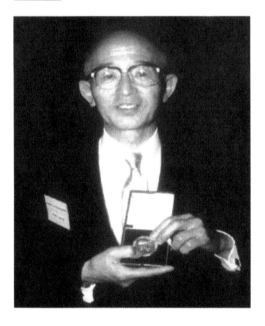

Photograph of Morio Kasai in May 1999.
(Kindly supplied by Professor Ryoji Ohi,
Miyagi Children's Hospital, Sendai, Japan)

Morio Kasai (1922–2008)

Morio Kasai was born on 19 September 1922 in the Aomori Prefecture in the northern part of Honshu, the main island in Japan. After graduating from Tohoku University School of Medicine in Sendai, he pursued a surgical career, specialising in paediatric surgery.

Until 1955, attempts to achieve bile drainage for 'uncorrectable' types of biliary atresia (90% of all cases) had failed. Construction of artificial bile ducts and lymphatic drainage of bile were just two of the unsuccessful techniques that had been tried. In 1955, Kasai's Chief of Surgery, Professor Shigetsugu Katsura operated on a 72-day-old girl whose extrahepatic bile ducts were completely occluded. Being unable to identify any patent extrahepatic bile ducts, Katsura incised the porta hepatis and sutured the duodenum over the area. The infant's jaundice subsequently resolved. In his next case, Katsura attached the unopened duodenum directly to the incised porta hepatis. Although this patient failed to clear their jaundice and subsequently died, some bile had been noticed in the infant's stool. At the autopsy, Kasai found a biliary fistula between the intrahepatic bile ducts and the duodenum. This was the starting point for developing and refining the Kasai portoenterostomy. The next infant in the Tohoku series underwent a planned hepatic portoenterostomy and the infant's jaundice resolved. Further histological studies in infants with biliary atresia showed the presence of patent microscopic bile ductules up to several hundred microns in size at the porta hepatis, even when the extrahepatic biliary tree was completely occluded.

Kasai first reported his new operative technique in an English language journal in 1968 but it took another 10 years for the procedure to be accepted in the West. Professor Ryoji Ohi, Kasai's successor, states that Kasai remarked that he had been able to proceed with his research unhurriedly because other paediatric surgeons hardly believed in his procedure!

Kasai succeeded Katsura and was appointed Professor and Chief of Surgery at Tokohu University Hospital in 1963, retiring in 1986. He continued to research biliary atresia and reported on the long-term outcome of his patients 20 or more years after portoenterostomy. In recognition of his achievements, Kasai was awarded the Denis Browne Gold Medal in Paediatric Surgery in 1986 and the Ladd Medal in 1991.

Not only was Kasai a pioneering paediatric surgeon but he also contributed to adult oesophageal cancer surgery through his work on perioperative surgical nutrition. He was a highly respected teacher and a great ambassador for Japanese paediatric surgery. He suffered a stroke in 1999, which restricted his activities, but he continued to enjoy his family. He died in December 2008.

References

Kasai M, Suzuki S. A new operation for 'non-correctable' biliary atresia: hepatic porto-enterostomy [in Japanese]. *Shujutsu* 1959;**13**:733–9.

Kasai M, Kimura S, Asakura Y, Suzuki H, Taira Y, Ohashi E. Surgical treatment of biliary atresia. *J Pediatr Surg* 1968;**3**:665–75.

Further reading

Kasai M, Ohi R, Chiba T et al. A patient with biliary atresia who died 28 years after hepatic portoenterostomy. *J Pediatr Surg* 1988;**23**:430–1.

Miyano T. Morio Kasai, MD, 1922–2008. *Pediatr Surg Int* 2009;25:307–8.

Ohi R. A history of the Kasai operation: hepatic portoenterostomy for biliary atresia. *World J Surg* 1988;**12**:871–4.

Ohi R. Pediatric surgery in Japan – past, present, and future. *J Pediatr Surg* 1996;**31**:305–9.

Klatskin tumour

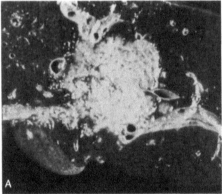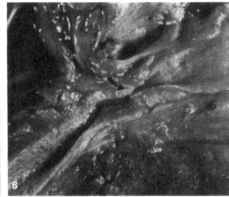

(A) Annular sclerosing adenocarcinoma at the bifurcation of the hepatic duct. (B) Bulky adenocarcinoma encircling and occluding the bifurcation of the common hepatic duct. (Reproduced with permission from Klatskin G. Adenocarcinoma of the hepatic duct at its bifurcation within the porta hepatis. An unusual tumor with distinctive clinical and pathological features. *Am J Med* 1965;**38**:241–56. Figs 1 & 2, p.251. © Elsevier)

In 1965, Klatskin highlighted the clinical features of cholangiocarcinoma at the bifurcation of the common hepatic duct in 13 patients. This is now known as a Klatskin tumour. In particular, he commented on the presentation with obstructive jaundice, potential for misdiagnosis at laparotomy, imaging appearances, pathology of the tumour, and effectiveness of palliative surgical biliary drainage.

Gerald Klatskin (1910–1986)

Gerald Klatskin was born in New York City to parents of Russian origin and graduated from Cornell University Medical School in 1929, first in his class. He began his association with Yale as an intern in 1933. During World War II, he served in the U.S Army as a medical officer in Calcutta, India, where the prevalence of hepatitis and amoebic abscess sparked his interest in liver disease. Returning to Yale in 1946, he established a renowned hepatology unit, eventually becoming Professor Emeritus in 1978.

Klatskin was an early pioneer of the technique of percutaneous liver biopsy. He performed the first at Yale in 1947 (Menghini reported his "one-second" aspiration technique in 1958) and even though the Pathology department made a fuss about the miserable size of the specimen, he persisted and, with the help of a talented laboratory technician, Hazel Hubbel, perfected the technique. Klatskin also contributed to the discovery of the link between 'Australia antigen' and hepatitis B and between alcohol-induced hyperlipidaemia and acute pancreatitis. He was one of the first to document the clinical significance of granulomas in the liver. However,

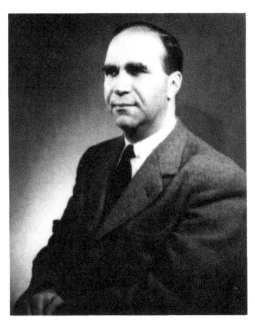

Gerald Klatskin (1949). (Courtesy of the National Library of Medicine)

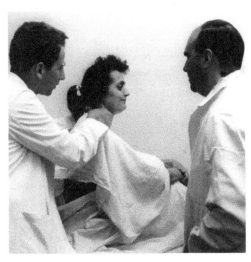

Dr Klatskin (right) with a patient. (Courtesy of Yale University, Harvey Cushing/John Hay Whitney Medical Library)

he is probably best remembered for his description of cholangiocarcinoma at the bifurcation of the common hepatic duct.

Affectionately called the "Klat" or "Great Bear", he was well known for his meticulous and detailed history taking and had an encyclopaedic knowledge of liver function and disease. In addition to his talents as a superb clinician and an outstanding liver pathologist, he was also an accomplished photographer. Over the years, he accumulated a collection of more than 50,000 colour slides from local

95

and referred liver biopsy specimens. For each sample in the collection, the history, physical findings, and laboratory results were recorded on one side of a file card and a detailed description of the histology on the other. His book on *Histopathology of the Liver* was started in the late 1970s but failing health and near-blindness prevented him completing the task, which was accomplished by Harold O. Conn. This seminal reference work was published posthumously in 1993.

Klatskin received numerous awards including the Francis Blake Award from Yale for outstanding teaching in medicine and the Julius Friedenwald medal from the American Gastroenterological Association. He was married to Ethelyn Elmer Henry, who became Professor Emeritus of Psychology and Pediatrics at the Yale Child Study Center. They had two daughters and a son.

References

Klatskin G. Adenocarcinoma of the hepatic duct at its bifurcation within the porta hepatis. An unusual tumor with distinctive clinical and pathological features. *Am J Med* 1965;**38**:241–56.

Klatskin G, Conn HO. *Histopathology of the Liver*. Oxford University Press, New York, 1993.

Menghini G. One-second needle biopsy of the liver. *Gastroenterology* 1958;**35**:190–199.

Further reading

Anon. Dr Gerald Klatskin is dead; authority on liver disorders. *New York Times*, March 30, 1986.

Boyer JL. Friedenwald presentation to Gerald Klatskin, M.D. *Gastroenterology* 1983;**85**:1235–8.

Kaplan M. Book review: Histopathology of the Liver. *N Engl J Med* 1994;**330**:148.

Klatskin G, Yesner R. Hepatic manifestations of sarcoidosis and other granulomatous diseases; a study based on histological examination of tissue obtained by needle biopsy of the liver. *Yale J Biol Med* 1950;**23**:207–48.

Myron L, Floch MH. 50 Years of Leadership of the Yale Digestive Disease Program. *J Clin Gastroenterol* 2005;**39**(Suppl 2):S29–32.

Yale University School of Medicine Dept of Internal Medicine website http://www.med.yale.edu/intmed/history/history_page_5.html (Last accessed 30 July 2007).

Kocher's incision/Kocher's manoeuvre

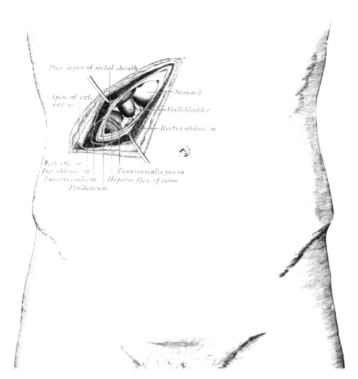

"Cholecystotomy – the incision here is for a difficult case. For a simple case, an incision is employed of half this length, the centre being over the edge of the rectus." (Adapted from Kocher T. *Textbook of Operative Surgery*. Translated from the 4th German edition by Harold J Stiles, Adam and Charles Black, London, 1903, p.227)

Kocher reported his subcostal incision for exposure of the gall bladder in 1890 (Liebermann–Meffert 2000). The technique of mobilising the second part of the duodenum by division of its lateral peritoneal attachments was described in 1903 (Kocher 1903). This procedure, now known as 'Kocherisation of the duodenum' or 'Kocher's manoeuvre', facilitated duodenal surgery and enabled better assessment of the head of the pancreas. However, Kocher was probably not the originator since the technique had previously been reported by a French surgeon in 1896 (Madden et al 1968).

Emil Theodor Kocher (1841–1917)

Kocher was born in Bern, Switzerland, the son of an engineer and a deeply religious Protestant mother. He graduated from the University of Bern in 1865. Anaesthesia had recently been publicly introduced by William Morton in 1846 and antisepsis by Joseph Lister in 1867. He studied with von Langenbeck and Virchow in Berlin, Billroth in Vienna, Spencer Wells and Lister in London, and Pasteur in Paris before being appointed to the Chair of Surgery at the University Hospital of Bern at just 31 years of age. Despite numerous tempting offers from around Europe, he remained in Bern for the rest of his career.

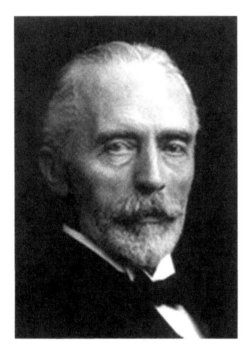

Theodor Kocher.

Kocher became a renowned Swiss surgeon by virtue of pioneering meticulous surgery, as well as devising numerous surgical techniques and instruments. These included Kocher's technique for reduction of a dislocated shoulder, Kocher's pedicle forceps, gland dissector and thyroid retractor, and Kocher's incision for thyroidectomy (in addition to the eponymous incision and manoeuvre described above).

Following in the Lister tradition, he was strict about asepsis and haemostasis, and, although a relatively slow operator, he was precise and careful. Kocher was quoted as saying: "Surgeons who take unnecessary risks and operate by the clock are exciting from the onlookers' standpoint but they are not necessarily those in whose hands you would choose to place yourself" (Rutkow 1978). As Moynihan stated, "… every operation Kocher ever did was a supreme exhibition of what perfect anatomical knowledge, a blameless aseptic conscience, the most practiced technical efficiency, unfaltering courage, unruffled calm, and the most exquisite gentleness could accomplish". From these comments, it comes as no surprise that Kocher was a perfectionist and a prized teacher. He developed close friendships with both

William Halsted at Johns Hopkins Hospital in Baltimore and the famous American neurosurgeon, Harvey Cushing.

Kocher was a pioneer in many branches of surgery including thyroidectomy (by March 1912 he had performed some 5000 operations for goitre, which was endemic in the iodine-deficient population of alpine Switzerland at that time);

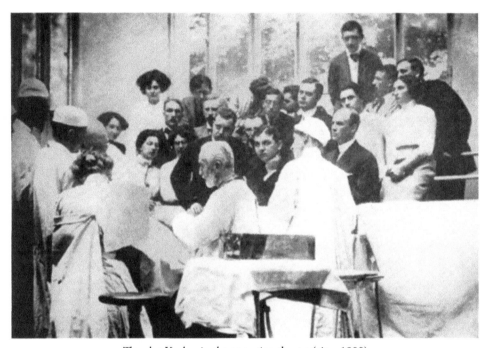

Theodor Kocher in the operating theatre (circa 1900)

oral surgery; abdominal surgery; trauma; and orthopaedics. He wrote extensively on abdominal surgery and surgical infections and was a great innovator in biliary tract surgery. He established the procedure for managing distal common bile duct stones by choledochoduodenostomy and, with a colleague, he reported a series of 100 operations on the bile ducts.

Kocher was widely celebrated as a surgical giant. He was a prolific writer and his textbook on operative surgery ran to many editions and was translated into several languages. He was an honorary member of the American Surgical Society, a member of the New York Academy of Medicine and the College of Physicians (Philadelphia), and an honorary fellow of the Royal College of Surgeons of England (1913). In 1902, he became President of the German Society of Surgeons in Berlin and, in 1905 he was President of the First International Surgical Congress in Brussels. Kocher became the first surgeon to be awarded the Nobel Prize in Physiology or Medicine in 1909, for his work on the physiology, pathology and surgery of the thyroid gland. In Bern,

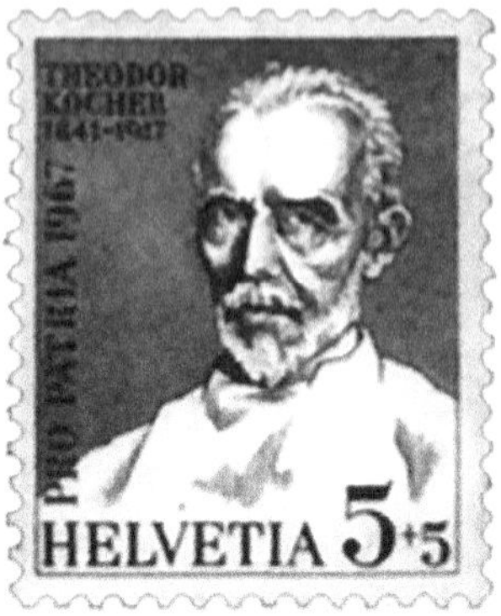

A Swiss postage stamp issued in 1967 to commemorate the 50th anniversary of Theodor Kocher's death.

a biomedical institute, a park and a street are named after him and in China there was even a volcano that bore his name (now called the Wudalianchi volcano).

Kocher married a Bernese merchant's daughter in 1869 and they had three sons, the eldest of whom, Albert, became Assistant Professor of Surgery and worked alongside his father. Whilst still in full time work, Theodor Kocher died unexpectedly from renal failure at the age of 76 years. Sir Berkeley Moynihan summed up the sentiments of the time with the comment: "With the death of Kocher, the world loses its greatest surgeon."

References

Kocher T. Mobilisierung des duodenum und gastroduodenostomie. *Zentralbl Chir* 1903;**30**:33–40.

Liebermann-Meffert DI. Short story of Theodor Kocher's life and relationship to the International Society of Surgery. *World J Surg* 2000;**24**:2–9.

Madden JL, Kandalaft S, Eghrari M. Mobilization of the duodenum: a surgical maneuver incorrectly credited to Kocher. *Surgery* 1968;**63**:522–526.

Rutkow IM. William Halsted and Theodor Kocher: "an exquisite friendship". *Ann Surg* 1978;**188**:630–7.

Further reading

Ellis H. *Bailey and Bishop's Notable Names in Medicine and Surgery.* 4th edition. H.K. Lewis & Co. Ltd, London, 1983, pp123–7.

Isepponi O, Huwiler V, Boschung U. Theodor Kocher's surgical and clinical case presentations. *Bull Hist Med* 2004;**78**:192–4.

Klebs AC. Theodor Kocher, 1841–1917. *U.S. Navy Medical Bulletin* 1918;**12**:59–63.

Kocher T, Matti H. Ueber Hundert Operationen an den Gallenwegen mit Bercksichtigung der Dauererfolge. *Archiv für Klinische Chirurgie* 1906;**81**:1–80.

McGreevy PS, Miller FA. Biography of Theodor Kocher. *Surgery* 1969;**65**:990–999.

The Nobel Foundation. *Nobel Lectures, Physiology or Medicine 1901–1921*, Elsevier Publishing Company, Amsterdam, 1967.

Wood M. Eponyms in biliary tract surgery. *Am J Surg* 1979;**138**:746–54.

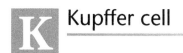

Kupffer cell

Ueber Sternzellen der Leber.

Briefliche Mittheilung an Prof. Waldeyer.

Von

C. Kupffer.

Title section of Kupffer's 1876 publication

Whilst Kupffer was working at the University of Kiel, he discovered these eponymous cells in the perisinusoidal space within the liver. In a letter to a fellow anatomist, Heinrich Waldeyer (1836–1921) in 1876, Carl von Kupffer commented on the cells he described as "Sternzellen" (star or stellate cells); no illustrations were provided in the letter (Kupffer 1876). He had found the cells serendipitously when using histological stains to search for nerve fibres. Initially he believed they were connective tissue cells but, from later experiments, Kupffer erroneously concluded that they were phagocytic endothelial cells.

In 1898, a Polish pathologist, Tadeusz Browicz (1847–1928), correctly identified the macrophages of the human liver sinusoids, later classified as part of the mononuclear phagocyte system and now called Kupffer cells. Subsequent ultrastructural studies showed that these were quite distinct from sinusoidal endothelial cells. The work of Kenjiro Wake and others from the early 1970s onwards showed that Kupffer's original stellate cells are neither endothelial cells nor phagocytic macrophages but are in fact perisinusoidal hepatic stellate cells, synonymous with Ito's fat-storing cells. Their lipid droplets are largely composed of retinoid (vitamin A) esters. They are contractile and regulate sinusoidal blood flow. They are also involved in collagen synthesis and have been found in other viscera. In the last 30 years their role in hepatic fibrosis and cirrhosis has been of particular interest.

Carl Wilhelm von Kupffer (1829–1902)

Carl Kupffer was a German anatomist who discovered the hepatic stellate cell. He was born in Lestene, in a region that is now part of Latvia, the first child of a pastor. Kupffer received his medical doctorate from the University of Tartu in 1854. After a brief period as a country doctor, he undertook postgraduate studies in Vienna, **101**

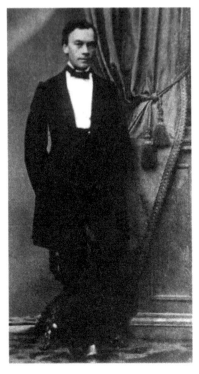

Carl von Kupffer. (Courtesy of the University of Tartu
Library, Tartu, Estonia. F78, Fo Norm 17:134)

Berlin and Göttingen. In 1858 he returned to Tartu, where he worked as a prosector
until 1865. Over the ensuing years, he held three consecutive university Chairs
of Anatomy: at the University of Kiel from 1867, at the University of Königsberg
between 1876 and 1880 and, from 1880 until his retirement in 1901, at the Ludwig
Maximilians University of Munich.

Kupffer is best known for his work in the fields of embryology, histology, and
comparative anatomy. He was particularly interested in the spinal cord, cranial
nerves, stomach and liver. During his time at the University of Königsberg, he had
the opportunity of studying the skull of the famous philosopher Immanuel Kant
(1724–1804), whose body was exhumed.

Although often referred to as Karl Kupffer, he signed himself 'Carl'. He married
in 1869 and had two children. He died of pneumonia after a stroke.

References

Kupffer C. Ueber Sternzellen der Leber. Briefliche mittheilung an Professor Waldeyer. *Arch Mikr Anat*
1876;**12**:353–8.

Further reading

Dean B. The seventieth birthday of Carl von Kupffer – his life and works. *Science* 1900;**11**:364–9.

Haines DE. The Contributors to Volume 1 (1891) of The Journal of Comparative Neurology: C.L. Herrick, C.H. Turner, H.R. Pemberton, B.G. Wilder, F.W. Langdon, C.J. Herrick, C. von Kupffer, O.S. Strong, T.B. Stowell. *J Comp Neurol* 1991;**314**:9–33.

Kupffer C, Bessel Hagen F. Der Schädel von Immanuel Kant. *Arch Anthropol* 1881;**13**:359–410.

Kupffer C. Über die sogennanten Sternzellen der Säugethierleber. *Arch Mikroskop Anat* 1899;**54**:254–88.

Wake K. Karl Wilhelm Kupffer and his contributions to modern hepatology. *Comp Hepatol* 2004;**3** (Suppl 1):S2. http://www.pubmedcentral.nih.gov/articlerender.fcgi?artid=2410225 (Last accessed December 2008).

Laennec's cirrhosis

DE

L'AUSCULTATION

MÉDIATE

ou

TRAITÉ DU DIAGNOSTIC DES MALADIES

DES POUMONS ET DU CŒUR,

FONDÉ PRINCIPALEMENT SUR CE NOUVEAU
MOYEN D'EXPLORATION.

Par R. T. H. LAENNEC,

D. M. P., Médecin de l'Hôpital Necker, Médecin honoraire
des Dispensaires, Membre de la Société de la Faculté de
Médecine de Paris et de plusieurs autres sociétés nationales
et étrangères.

Μέγα δὲ μέρος ἡγεῦμαι τῆς τέχνης εἶναι
τὸ δύνασθαι σκοπεῖν.

Pouvoir explorer est, à mon avis, une
grande partie de l'art. Hipp., *Epid. III*.

TOME PREMIER.

A PARIS,

Chez J.-A. BROSSON et J.-S. CHAUDÉ, Libraires,
rue Pierre-Sarrazin, nº 9.

1819.

Title page of Laennec's treatise in which the term 'cirrhosis' was first used

The French physician, René Laennec coined the term 'cirrhosis' from the Greek word *kirrhos* (meaning tawny) because of the tawny yellow-coloured nodules seen in affected livers. This reference first appeared as a footnote to the postmortem findings on a 47-year-old ex-soldier, Jean Edme, who Laennec reported in the first edition of his famous treatise *De l'Auscultation Médiate* published in 1819 (Laennec 1819). A description of cirrhosis had been published previously by John Browne (1642–1702), a seventeenth century English surgeon and anatomist (Browne 1685). Matthew Baillie (1762–1823), an anatomist and physician at St George's Hospital in London, and a correspondent with Laennec had made the link between alcohol and cirrhosis but Laennec seems to have been unaware of this. In an unpublished *Treatise of Pathological Anatomy* written between 1804 and 1808, Laennec expanded on his description of what we would now call micronodular cirrhosis of the liver (Duffin 1987). He did not speculate on the cause of the condition. Furthermore, he erroneously included a few other entities such as cystic disease of the liver within the spectrum of cirrhosis.

105

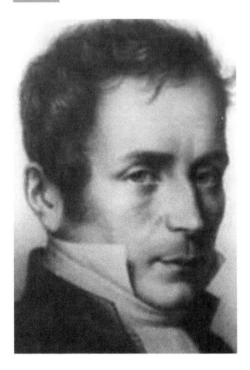

René Théophile Hyacinthe Laennec.

René Théophile Hyacinthe Laennec (1781–1826)

Laennec was chief physician at the Necker Hospital in Paris from 1816. It was here that he invented the stethoscope. He described how, when faced with an overweight young woman with suspected heart disease, percussion and palpation of the chest were useless on account of her obesity, and modesty precluded direct auscultation. So, using a rolled up sheet of paper as an ear trumpet, he listened to her heart sounds. Based on his subsequent experience with wooden stethoscopes, he published his famous treatise on auscultation (*De l'Auscultation Médiate*) in 1819.

In 1822, Laennec was appointed as Professor of Medicine at the Collège de France and the following year he became Professor at the Hôpital de la Charité and was elected to the Académie de Médecine. Other notable academic contributions included a seminal work on tuberculosis (although he did not realise that this was an infectious disease) and a description of pulmonary metastases from malignant melanoma. He also coined the term melanoma (he actually used the term 'melanose' from the Greek *mela* for black). His penchant for Greek terms stemmed from having studied the classics, partly in order to be able to read the original writings of Hippocrates and others.

Throughout his life, Laennec was a devout Catholic. He died from tuberculosis at the age of 45 years. He has been the subject of several biographies. Among the

106

various tributes to his life are a memorial tablet outside the Hôpital Necker Enfants Malades in Paris, a bronze statue in the town of Quimper in Brittany, where he was born, and a museum in Nantes. He was commemorated on a French postage stamp in 1952.

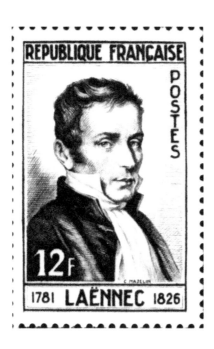

References

Browne J. A remarkable account of a liver, appearing glandulous to the eye. *Philos Trans R Soc* 1685;**15**:1266–8.

Duffin JM. Why does cirrhosis belong to Laennec? *CMAJ* 1987;**137**:393–6.

Laennec RTH. *De l'Auscultation Médiate ou Traité du Diagnostic des Maladies des Poumons et du Coeur, Fondé Principalement sur ce Nouveau Moyen d'Exploration*. Volume 1: JA Brosson et JS Chaudé. Paris, 1819, pp359–69.

Further reading

Denkler K, Johnson J. A lost piece of melanoma history. *Plast Reconstr Surg* 1999;**104**:2149–53.

Kervran R. *Laennec: his life and times*. Pergamon Press, London, 1959.

Islets of Langerhans

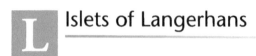

Beiträge
zur mikroskopischen Anatomie der
Bauchspeicheldrüse.

INAUGURAL-DISSERTATION,

ZUR

ERLANGUNG DER DOCTORWÜRDE

IN DER

MEDICIN UND CHIRURGIE

VORGELEGT DER

MEDICINISCHEN FACULTÄT

DER FRIEDRICH-WILHELMS-UNIVERSITÄT

ZU BERLIN

UND ÖFFENTLICH ZU VERTHEIDIGEN

am 18. Februar 1869

VON

Paul Langerhans

aus Berlin.

OPPONENTEN:

O. Loeillot de Mars, Dd. med.
O. Soltmann, Dd med.
Paul Ruge, Stud. med.

BERLIN.

BUCHDRUCKEREI VON GUSTAV LANGE

Title page of Langerhans' 1869 thesis on the microscopic anatomy of the pancreas

In the introduction to his 31-page MD thesis presented in 1869 entitled *Beiträge zur mikroskopischen Anatomie der Bauchspeicheldrüse* (Contributions on the Microscopic Anatomy of the Pancreas), Langerhans stated: "There is hardly another organ in which such a glaring contrast exists between the brilliant results of physiological research and the complete darkness in the realm of anatomical knowledge". He went on to provide the first description of pancreatic islets based on histological observations made on pancreatic tissue from a variety of animals, including the salamander, rabbit and man. Langerhans recognised clusters of small irregularly polygonal cells with clear cytoplasm diffusely scattered throughout the gland, each measuring 0.1–0.24 mm in diameter. Unfortunately, there are no drawings of these cell clusters in his thesis. He did not know or suggest the function of these cells and it is likely that he and his mentors did not appreciate their significance. Langerhans was apologetic about these results: "With regret, I must begin my communication with the declaration that I cannot in any way put forth the conclusive results of a completed investigation. I can describe, at most, a few isolated observations which suggest a much more complicated structure of the organ [pancreas] than hitherto accepted." It was not until 1893, some 24 years later, that the French histopathologist Edouard Laguesse (1861–1927) suggested that the "islets of Langerhans" were the site of an internal secretion of the pancreas later named insulin.

Although the pancreas had been studied since the 16th century, up to the time of Langerhans' discovery only the secretory acini and ductal system were known about and the organ was classified anatomically as a salivary gland, as indicated by the term *Bauchspeicheldrüse*. Langerhans began the experimental work for his doctoral thesis in the summer of 1867 but his research was interrupted three months later, when he competed for the Berlin University faculty prize in medicine. He won the prize (and 25 gold ducats) for his investigation of the tactile corpuscles in the skin. After returning to his research on the pancreas in October 1868, he completed the project in just six months.

The year after Langerhan's death, von Mering and Minkowski reported that diabetes could be induced experimentally in dogs by pancreatectomy and, in 1901 Eugene Opie noted the link between pathology of the islets and diabetes mellitus. Insulin was discovered by Charles Herbert Best (1899–1978) and Frederick Grant Banting (1891–1941) in Toronto in 1921.

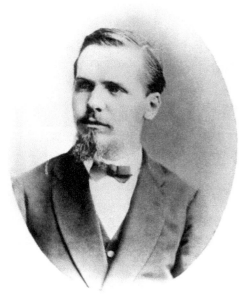

Paul Langerhans. (© Bildarchiv Preußischer Kulturbesitz, Berlin, 1873. Photographer: Ruf und Dilger)

Paul Langerhans (1847–1888)

Langerhans was born in Berlin, the son of a successful physician. His mother died of tuberculosis when he was six years old. He had two half brothers from his father's second marriage, both of whom became physicians. Paul Wilhelm Heinrich Langerhans began his medical studies at the University of Jena in 1865, where he was influenced by the eminent biologist, Ernst Haeckel (1834–1919). He then transferred to the University of Berlin, where he was a student of the famous pathologist, Rudolf Virchow (1821–1902), who was also a family friend.

Langerhans was an exceedingly gifted and industrious medical student. Not only was he the first to identify pancreatic islets but he also made two other important discoveries as a student. Whilst at the Berlin Pathological Institute in 1867, Langerhans discovered dendritic cells in the skin (later known as Langerhans cells). He initially thought these were cutaneous nervous system receptors but they are now known to be antigen-presenting cells of the macrophage system involved in cell-mediated immunity. Clonal proliferation of these cells is the basis of the spectrum of disorders known as Langerhans cell histiocytosis. In the same paper, he also described the granular cells of the stratum granulosum in the epidermis.

After graduation, Langerhans worked in Virchow's laboratory for a further year and then, in 1870, he joined an expedition to the Middle East, where he undertook some medical and anthropological studies. During the Franco–Prussian War (1870–1871) he served as a medical officer in the Prussian army in Germany and France. After the war, he became Prosector in Pathology at the University of Frieburg, where he continued his histological studies. At just 27 years of age, he was appointed to a Chair but within weeks of this promotion he was diagnosed as having pulmonary tuberculosis. This not only forced him to give up the position but prompted his search for a cure in Switzerland, Italy and Germany.

In 1875, Langerhans settled in Madeira, where the climate was considered beneficial to his health. He began an entirely new area of research, studying marine worms. The fact that he described more than 50 new species is further testimony to his capacity for hard work and critical observation, for which he was rewarded with a grant of 2000 gold marks from the Berlin Academy of Sciences. A year after arriving in Madeira, Langerhans became free from fever, only to experience a relapse when he briefly returned to Jena in 1878. Subsequently he returned to Madeira, where he recovered to the extent that he began practicing medicine, caring for German and British immigrants to the island (also mostly suffering from tuberculosis). In addition to his diverse academic interests, he wrote a famous guidebook to Madeira.

In June 1885, during one of several brief trips to Berlin, Paul Langerhans married a widow, Margarethe Ebart. Together with Margarethe's daughter they shared three happy years. On 20 July 1888, just days before his 41st birthday, Langerhans died from chronic renal failure secondary to renal tuberculosis. He was buried in the British cemetery at Funchal in Madeira. On his gravestone is an epitaph written in Greek taken from Homer's *Odyssey*, which Langerhans translated as "Nor did he wish to live any longer nor to see the light of the beaming sun".

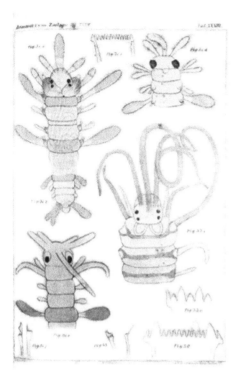

A plate showing original drawings of marine worms by Langerhans. The top left figure shows the head and tail of the asexual form of Virchowia clavata, a new genus and species of annelid worm discovered by Langerhans and named in honour of his previous mentor. (From Langerhans P. Die Wurmfauna von Madeira. Zeitschrift fur Wissenschaftliche Zoologie 1879;32:513–92, Taf. XXXIII, Figs 31–33)

References

Langerhans P. *Beiträge zur mikroskopischen Anatomie der Bauchspeicheldrüse.* MD dissertation, Berlin, Gustav Lange, 1869.

Langerhans P. Die Wurmfauna von Madeira. I. *Z Wiss Zool* 1879;**32**:513–92.

Further reading

Barach JH. Paul Langerhans 1847–1888. *Diabetes* 1952;**1**:411–3.

Campbell WR. Paul Langerhans, 1847–1888. *Can Med Assoc J* 1958;**79**:855–6.

Ebling FJ. Homage to Paul Langerhans. *J Invest Dermatol* 1980;**75**:3–5.

Egeler RM, Zantinga AR, Coppes M. Paul Langerhans Jr. (1847–1888): a short life, yet two eponymic legacies. *Med Pediatr Oncol* 1994;**22**:129–32.

Giacometti L, Barss M. Paul Langerhans: a tribute. *Arch Dermatol* 1969;**100**:770–2.

Hausen BM. The man behind the eponym. Paul Langerhans – life and work. Part I. Childhood, early education, and college education. *Am J Dermatopathol* 1987;**9**:151–6.

Hausen BM. The man behind the eponym. Paul Langerhans – life and work. Part II. Postgraduate studies, travels, first signs of disease, Madeira. *Am J Dermatopathol* 1987;**9**:157–62.

Hausen BM. The man behind the eponym. Paul Langerhans. Life and work. Part III: Scientific research, marriage, and death. *Am J Dermatopathol* 1987;**9**:264–9.

111

Hausen BM. Paul Langerhans. Life and work. Part IV: Publications. *Am J Dermatopathol* 1987;**9**:270–5.

Hausen BM. *Die Inseln des Paul Langerhans. Eine Biographie in Bildern und Dokumenten.* Ueberreuter Wissenschafts Verlag, Vienna, 1988.

Langerhans P. Zur pathologischen Anatomie der Tastkörper. *Virch Arch Pathol Anat* 1869;**45**:413–17.

Morrison H. *Contributions to the Microscopic Anatomy of the Pancreas.* By Paul Langerhans (Berlin, 1869). Reprint of the German original with an English translation and an introductory essay. *Bull Inst Hist Med* 1937;**5**:259–97.

Sakula A. Paul Langerhans (1847–1888): a centenary tribute. *J R Soc Med* 1988;**81**:414–5.

LeVeen peritoneo-venous shunt

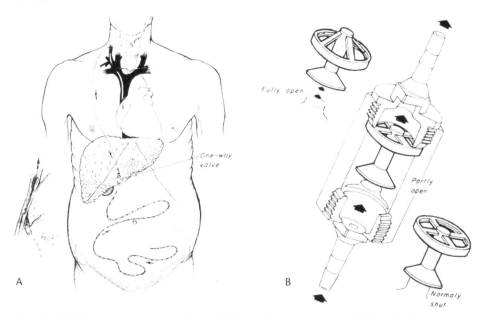

A   B

The original LeVeen peritoneo-venous shunt (A). The valve (B) is normally held in the closed position by tension on the silicone rubber struts. (From LeVeen HH, Christoudias G, Moon IP, Luft R, Falk G, Grosberg S. Peritoneo-venous shunting for ascites. *Ann Surg* 1974;180:580–91, Fig. 6, p.584 and Fig. 2, p.581. © Lippincott, Williams & Wilkins)

The LeVeen shunt is a silicone tube that passes subcutaneously from the peritoneal cavity to the superior vena cava by way of the jugular vein. A pressure-sensitive one-way disc valve permits the flow of ascitic fluid into the venous circulation when the intraperitoneal pressure exceeds the intrathoracic venous pressure by 3–5 cm water. The concept was not new but the design of the device was. Cyclical changes in intrathoracic pressure with respiration and the prevention of reflux of blood into the tubing were critical factors. Experimental testing of the LeVeen shunt began in dogs in 1972 and the device was then used in patients. In their 1974 publication, LeVeen and colleagues reported outcomes in 45 patients who had the shunt inserted for cirrhotic ascites, 28 of whom experienced symptomatic relief for up to 18 months (LeVeen et al 1974). Although the shunt was designed to drain non-malignant ascites, it was later used as a palliative intervention in patients with malignant ascites.

At around the same time that LeVeen and colleagues reported their results, the Denver shunt was introduced. This was designed by John Newkirk, an engineer at Denver University, and was initially applied to the treatment of hydrocephalus (Kirsch et al 1970). This shunt had a subcutaneous manually compressible silicone pumping chamber containing a unidirectional pressure-activated valve; valve opening occurred at a pressure of only 1 cm water and, unlike the LeVeen shunt, patency of the shunt could be tested by percutaneous palpation. At first, the Denver shunt was used to treat patients with malignant ascites and drainage was to the inferior vena cava via the long saphenous vein (Waddell, discussion in LeVeen et al 1974). Results of its use in draining cirrhotic ascites via the jugular vein were not reported until 1979 (Lund and Newkirk 1979).

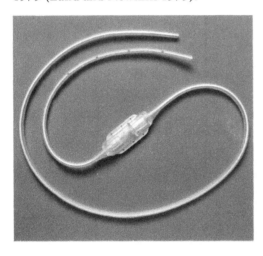

Denver shunt. (Cardinalhealth 2009)

Complications associated with both the LeVeen and Denver shunts occur in up to 40% of patients, particularly in patients with malignant disease (Lund and Moritz 1982). These include mechanical failure (kinking of the tube, valve occlusion by fibrin, ascitic leak at the insertion site), haemodilution, circulatory volume overload, electrolyte disturbances, disseminated intravascular coagulation, sepsis and central vein thrombosis. In one small randomised, controlled trial, the LeVeen shunt was found to have a better patency rate than the Denver shunt in patients with cirrhotic ascites (Fulenwider et al 1986) but both shunts have their advocates.

Peritoneo-venous shunts are less often used to treat cirrhotic ascites today because of the availability of better therapies such as transjugular intrahepatic portosystemic stent shunts (TIPS) and liver transplantation. However, they still have a selective role in the palliative treatment of malignant ascites and in the management of other causes of intractable ascites.

Harry Henry LeVeen (1914–1996)

Harry LeVeen was an American surgeon. Born in New York, he graduated from Princeton University in 1936 and obtained his medical degree from New York University College of Medicine in 1940. He undertook his residency training in centres in Jamaica, Long Island and Chicago. He was Professor of Surgery at the State University of New York and Chief of Surgery at what is now the Veterans Affairs Medical Center in Brooklyn. It was here in the 1970s that he devised the

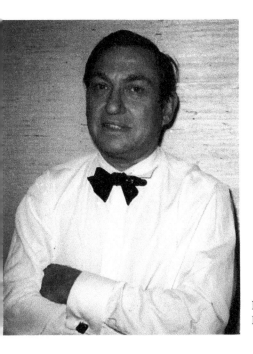

Harry LeVeen in 1970. (Kindly supplied by Dr Robert LeVeen)

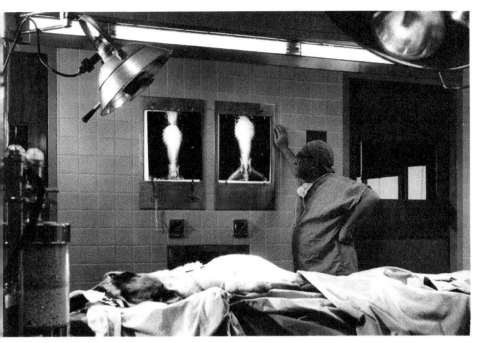

Harry LeVeen in the animal laboratory circa 1960. (Courtesy of Dr Robert LeVeen)

LeVeen shunt. In 1979, he became Chief of Surgery at the Medical University of South Carolina.

LeVeen's major areas of research included liver disease and vascular surgery. He wrote over 200 scientific articles and was awarded more than 100 patents for items ranging from medical devices to chemical processes. He was a fellow of the American College of Surgeons, the Royal Society of Medicine and the Royal College of Surgeons of England. After retiring in 1988 he continued his research; at the time of his death from heart failure he was working on bactericidal plastics, oral vaccines, and novel cancer therapies. Harry LeVeen was married with two sons, both of whom became physicians.

References

Fulenwider JT, Galambos JD, Smith RB 3rd, Henderson JM, Warren WD. LeVeen vs Denver peritoneovenous shunts for intractable ascites of cirrhosis. A randomized, prospective trial. *Arch Surg* 1986;**121**:351–5.

Kirsch WM, Newkirk JB, Predecki PK. Clinical experience with the Denver shunt: a new silicone rubber shunting device for the treatment of hydrocephalus. *J Neurosurg* 1970;**32**:258–64.

LeVeen HH, Christoudias G, Moon IP, Luft R, Falk G, Grosberg S. Peritoneo-venous shunting for ascites. *Ann Surg* 1974;**180**:580–91.

Lund RH, Moritz MW. Complications of Denver peritoneovenous shunting. *Arch Surg* 1982;**117**:924–8.

Lund RH, Newkirk JB. Peritoneo-venous shunting system for surgical management of ascites. *Contemp Surg* 1979;**14**:31–45.

Further reading

Anon. Harry Henry LeVeen '36. Princeton University Archives. http://www.princeton.edu/~paw/archive_old/PAW96-97/14-0416/0416mem.html (Last accessed January 2009).

Burkhart F. Harry H. LeVeen, a Surgeon and Innovator, is Dead at 82. *New York Times* January 7, 1997.

LeVeen HH. The peritoneovenous shunt. Inception to maturity. *ASAIO Trans* 1990;**36**:50–5.

Lilly's technique for choledochal cyst excision

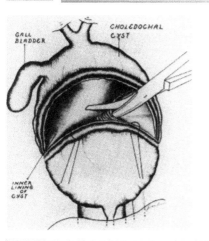

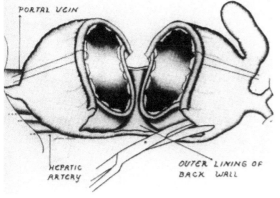

Drawings illustrating Lilly's technique for choledochal cyst excision. (Reproduced from Lilly JR. The surgical treatment of choledochal cyst. *Surg Gynecol Obstet* 1979;149:36–42 [now Journal of American College of Surgeons]. With permission of Elsevier)

When Lilly published his technique of surgical excision of choledochal cyst, radical cyst excision and reconstruction by hepaticoenterostomy was not routinely performed. Despite the recognised complications, treatment by internal drainage of the cyst into the duodenum or jejunum was still common. One reason for the reluctance to adopt cyst excision was the morbidity and mortality associated with the procedure. In 1978, Lilly first published his technique of choledochal cyst excision (Lilly 1978). In this procedure, the cyst is opened transversely across its anterior and lateral aspects and a plane of dissection is developed between the inner and outer layers of the posterior wall of the cyst. In this way, the thick inner lining of the choledochal cyst is excised but the thinner outer layer of the posterior wall of the cyst is retained, thereby minimising injury to the portal vein and hepatic artery, which are commonly adherent to the posterior wall of the cyst, particularly after previous inflammation or surgery. The distal common bile duct is suture ligated and the full thickness of the common hepatic duct is transected proximally. In his 1979 paper, Lilly reported successful cyst excision and Roux-en-Y reconstruction in nine of 11 children with a choledochal cyst, six of whom had had previous unsuccessful

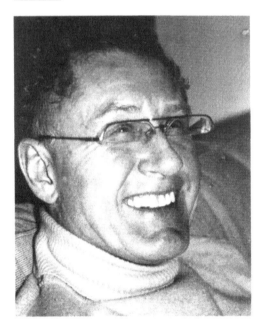

John Lilly. (Courtesy of Professor R. Peter Altman, New York)

surgery (Lilly 1979). The technique is rarely used today partly because most children are treated by definitive primary surgery at an early age before the onset of dense inflammatory adhesions and portal hypertension.

John Russell Lilly (1929–1995)

John Lilly was born in Milwaukee, Wisconsin. He was Dr Judson Randolph's first resident at the Children's Hospital in Washington, DC, where he contributed to building one of the foremost paediatric surgical services in the USA. In 1969, he moved to the University of Colorado at Denver, where he worked as Surgical Research Fellow in Transplantation with Dr Thomas Starzl, later becoming Surgeon-in-Chief at the Children's Hospital.

Lilly made many contributions to paediatric surgery, not least in paediatric hepatobiliary surgery. By all accounts he was a bold and innovative surgeon, a stimulating teacher, and a talented editor. According to Dr Peter Altman, one of Lilly's former residents and now Surgeon-in-Chief at the Morgan Stanley Children's Hospital at the New York Presbyterian Hospital, Columbia University Medical Center, New York, his fireside chats with trainees were legendary. He was as likely to recite extracts from Alice in Wonderland or ask residents to name the seven dwarfs as he was to question them on surgical principles!

Lilly was married twice and had three children.

References

Lilly JR. Total excision of choledochal cyst. *Surg Gynecol Obstet* 1978;**146**:254–6.

Lilly JR. The surgical treatment of choledochal cyst. *Surg Gynecol Obstet* 1979;**149**:36–42.

Further reading

Altman RP. Dr John Lilly Obituary. *Pediatr Surg Int* 1995;**10**:590.

L Longmire's intrahepatic cholangiojejunostomy

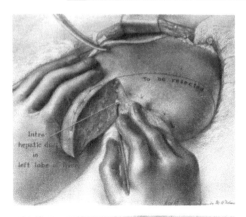

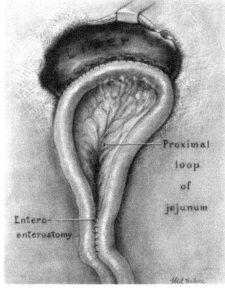

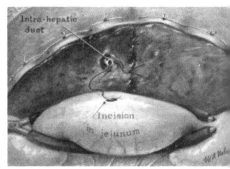

Division of the liver and identification of the dilated left intrahepatic duct (top left). Cholangioenterostomy with interrupted fine silk sutures over a small rubber catheter (right). Completed anastomosis with enteroenterostomy (bottom left). (Reprinted from Longmire WP Jr and Sanford MC. Intrahepatic cholangiojejunostomy with partial hepatectomy for biliary obstruction. *Surgery* 1948;24:264–76. With permission © Elsevier)

It was the problem of biliary atresia that prompted Longmire to develop th technique of partial hepatectomy and intrahepatic cholangiojejunostomy for biliar obstruction. In 1948, he proposed this as a useful method for treating biliar obstruction due to complex, benign, proximal common bile duct strictures. Whe Longmire devised this operation intrahepatic anatomy was poorly described, live transplantation had yet to be developed, and for most affected infants, biliary atresi was a death sentence.

After initially demonstrating the feasibility of the procedure in dogs, Longmire performed the first intrahepatic cholangiojejunostomy in April 1947. The patient was a 54-year-old woman with biliary cirrhosis secondary to a strictured choledochojejunostomy following a previous failed repair of a bile duct stricture. After excising the left lateral segment, he anastomosed a dilated intrahepatic bile duct to a jejunal loop. The patient's jaundice was relieved and she was reported to be reasonably well 9 months later. He then attempted the operation in three infants with biliary atresia but was unsuccessful because no dilated intrahepatic bile ducts could be found.

Longmire accepted that there were few indications for the technique (he had performed only nine such procedures by 1956) and that conventional biliary reconstruction should be attempted first. One advantage of his procedure was that the operative field avoided the scarred and distorted porta hepatis. In 1972, McArthur and Longmire reported an additional indication for intrahepatic cholangiojejunostomy, namely biliary decompression in patients with benign biliary strictures associated with portal hypertension (McArthur and Longmire 1972). Intrahepatic cholangiojejunostomy avoided the hazardous venous collaterals at the porta hepatis. Longmire stressed that success depended on the presence of dilated intrahepatic bile ducts free of obstructing debris, and adequate cross-communication between the right- and left-sided intrahepatic ducts.

Longmire's intrahepatic cholangiojejunostomy operation is rarely, if ever, performed these days because of safer hepaticojejunostomy techniques, such as the Hepp–Couinaud approach to the left hepatic duct (see Couinaud); endoscopic and interventional radiological techniques; and, in those with end-stage liver disease, transplantation.

William Polk Longmire Jr (1913–2003)

William Longmire was born in the rural town of Sapulpa, Oklahoma, where his father was a country doctor and his mother a schoolteacher. He graduated from the University of Oklahoma and obtained his MD from the Johns Hopkins University in Baltimore in 1938. His training was then interrupted when his father suffered a stroke. Longmire had to return home to maintain his father's practice. He later commented that this period in family practice was one of the most rewarding experiences of his training years.

After rejoining the surgical residency programme at Johns Hopkins, he became Alfred Blalock's (1899–1964) Chief Resident and assisted him with the first successful 'blue baby' operation in November 1944; this palliative operation for tetralogy of Fallot later became famous as the Blalock–Taussig shunt. Longmire excelled at general and thoracic surgery. Toward the end of his appointment at Johns Hopkins, he became known as the "Professor of Difficult Surgery"! No thoracic appointment

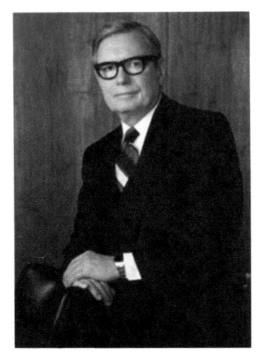

Dr William P. Longmire. (Courtesy of the
Longmire Surgical Society, David Geffen
School of Medicine, UCLA)

was available after he completed his residency in 1948, so he took up the post of
Associate Professor in charge of plastic surgery. In that same year a new medical
school at the University of California Los Angeles was being established. At the age
of 34 years, Longmire became the first Chairman of Surgery at UCLA, a position he
occupied with great distinction until 1976.

During his career he became President of the American College of Surgeons
and the American Surgical Association, and Chairman of the American Board of
Surgery. He was awarded honorary fellowships by the Royal College of Surgeons
of Edinburgh, England, and Ireland, and honorary degrees from the Universities
of Lund, Heidelberg, and Athens. In 1985 he had the distinction of being the first
honorary foreign member of the Japanese Surgical Society. In addition to a glittering
career in surgery, Longmire served in the US Air Force in the 1950s, rising to the
rank of major and later acting as Consultant to the Surgeon General.

Like many great surgeons, Longmire was recognised as a superb teacher, a skilled
operator and an outstanding academic, qualities that led to his reputation as an
internationally acclaimed surgical leader. He published more than 300 scientific
articles and four books (including a biography of Alfred Blalock). As well as
hepatobiliary techniques, he pioneered coronary endarterectomy (before the days
of routine coronary angiography), jejunal interposition after total gastrectomy, and
pylorus-preserving pancreaticoduodenectomy.

Longmire was married with two daughters, one of whom also qualified as a surgeon. He died in May 2003 after a two-decade struggle with a carcinoid tumour.

References

Longmire WP Jr, Sanford MC. Intrahepatic cholangiojejunostomy with partial hepatectomy for biliary obstruction. *Surgery* 1948;**24**:264–76.

McArthur MS, Longmire WP Jr. Further indications for intrahepatic cholangiojejunostomy. *Ann Surg* 1972;**175**:190–2.

Further reading

Hanlon CR. William Polk Longmire, Jr., MD, FACS, 1913–2003, remembered. *Bull Am Coll Surg* 2003;**88**:36–7.

Longmire WP Jr. Hepaticojejunostomy for biliary obstruction. *Rev Surg* 1971;**28**:385–90.

Longmire WP Jr: *Alfred Blalock: His Life and Times*. Privately published, Baltimore, 1991.

Mulder DG. In memoriam. University of California. http://www.universityofcalifornia.edu/senate/inmemoriam/WilliamP.LongmireJr..htm (Last accessed October 2007).

Traverso LW. The Longmire I, II, and III operations. *Am J Surg* 2003;**185**:399–406.

William P Longmire Jr. Recollections. http://www.williamlongmire.org/recollections.htm#Muller (Last accessed November 2007).

Cystic lymph node of Lund

Lymph from the gall bladder usually drains directly to intrahepatic lymphatics and into a single and prominent cystic node (the lymph node of Lund), which lies above the cystic duct in Calot's triangle. This cystic node is also sometimes referred to as Calot's node (see Calot). Efferent vessels from this lymph node pass to nodes in the free edge of the lesser omentum, where they communicate with lymph nodes at the hilum of the liver and coeliac lymph nodes. According to several sources, the lymph node of Lund was named after the American surgeon Fred Bates Lund but it has not yet been possible to trace his original description.

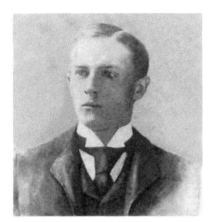 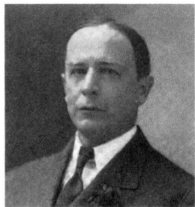

Fred Bates Lund as a Harvard medical student in 1888 (left) and 25 years later as a surgeon at Boston City Hospital (right). From Harvard College Class of 1888: Twenty-Fifth Anniversary Report. June, 1913. (By kind permission of Harvard University Archives, call # HUD 288.25)

Fred Bates Lund (1865–1950)

Lund was a surgeon at Boston City Hospital (now Boston University Medical Center) in the United States. He was born in Concord, New Hampshire, and obtained his MD from Harvard University in 1892. During his early years of surgical practice he also taught anatomy and lectured in surgery at Harvard Medical School. In 1926, he moved from being Surgeon-in-Chief at Boston City Hospital to become Surgeon-in-Chief at Carney Hospital in Boston, retiring in 1935. As a member of the American Society of Clinical Surgery (and later its president), Lund made several trips to Europe to visit the clinics of other surgeons. He also had an active military career, rising from the rank of major in the Harvard medical unit attached to the British Expeditionary Force in France in the First World War, to lieutenant colonel in the US Army Medical Reserve Corps.

He was a founder member and president of the American Surgical Association and an active member of the New York Surgical Society. Lund was a true general surgeon and published on a wide range of surgical topics including carotid body tumours, gallstone ileus, chest wall sarcoma, urology, and orthopaedics. He was also a classics scholar, and wrote books on Greek Medicine (1936) and Galen (1941), and articles on Hippocrates, Socrates, Plato, and Aristotle. He was married with five children, a daughter who sadly died in childhood and four boys.

References

Fred Bates Lund. Harvard College Class of 1888. Twenty-Fifth Anniversary Report. 1913, pp102–3.

Lund FB. *Greek Medicine.* Hoeber, New York, 1936.

Lund FB. *Galen on malingering, centaurs, diabetes and other subjects more or less related.* Columbia University Press, 1941.

Further reading

Anon. Lund, Fred Bates. *The National Cyclopaedia of American Biography.* Volume 46. University Microfilms, Ann Arbor, Michigan, 1967.

Fred Bates Lund. Harvard College Class of 1888. Fiftieth Anniversary Report. Cambridge, 1938, pp213–14.

Lund C. Fred Bates Lund, 1865–1950. *Transactions of the Meeting of the American Surgical Association* 1951;**96**:510–12.

Lund FB. The life and writings of Hippocrates. *Boston Med Surg J* 1924;**191**:1009–14.

Lund FB. The influence of the New York Surgical Society on the development of surgery. *Ann Surg* 1930;**91**:3–12.

Lund FB. Hippocratic Surgery. *Ann Surg* 1935;**102**:531–47.

Luschka's duct

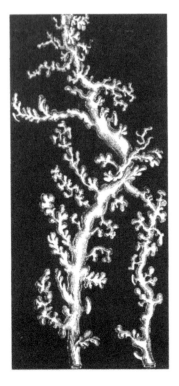

Bile ducts with glandular appendices from the left posterior longitudinal furrow of the human liver (50 times magnified). Although this is not Luschka's duct, it is a good example of Luschka's detailed investigation of gross biliary anatomy. (From Luschka H. Die Anatomie des menschlichen Bauches, Tübingen. Verlag der H Lauppschen, Buchhandlung, 1863, p.254, Fig. 35. By kind permission of the University of Tübingen Library [call number Jb I 278 b-2,1])

In 1863, Luschka first described a small bile duct passing from the gall bladder fossa in the right lobe of the liver connecting to the right hepatic duct or its anterior sectoral branch or the common hepatic duct. This subvesical duct typically drains a variable part of segment V of the liver but can drain posterior segments of the right liver. Rarely, it opens into the left hepatic duct, common bile duct or cystic duct. The importance of Luschka's duct is that it may be injured during cholecystectomy and cause a postoperative bile leak. Postmortem histological studies have found Luschka duct(s) in up to 30% of individuals but many of these are small and relatively insignificant. If larger ducts (1–2 mm) are considered, the incidence is nearer to 5%. These ducts are more likely to be injured if the gall bladder is not dissected close to its wall.

Luschka did not describe a duct communicating with the gall bladder (cystohepatic duct), which some authors have included within the definition.

Hubert von Luschka (1820–1875)

Born in the lakeside town of Konstanz (Constance) in southern Germany, where his father was a forest manager, Luschka was the eighth of 12 sons. He initially studied pharmacy but then transferred to medicine, moving to the University of Freiburg

126

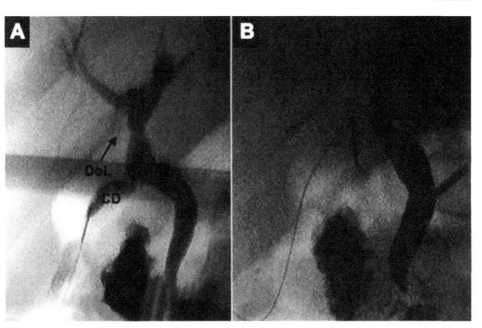

Operative cholangiogram performed at cholecystectomy for pigment gallstones (A) and at reoperation for bile leak (B) in a 12-year-old boy. The duct of Luschka (DoL) is marked by an arrow and was cannulated for the cholangiogram in B. CD, cystic duct. (Courtesy of Professor Jean de Ville de Goyet)

in 1841. He pursued his studies in Heidelberg (1843–1844), passing the state examination in Karlsruhe in 1844, and receiving his doctorate at Freiburg in 1845. Following a period as assistant to the German orthopaedic surgeon, Louis Stromeyer (1804–1876), Luschka undertook further studies in Paris, Vienna, and Northern Italy. In 1849 he was invited to Tübingen where, on the retirement of his former teacher, Friedrich Arnold (1803–1890), he was appointed to the Chair of Anatomy (1853), later becoming director of the prestigious Department of Anatomy. He occupied this position until his death.

Luschka is regarded as one of the foremost anatomists of the nineteenth century, and was a particularly distinguished gross anatomist. He was a prolific writer, contributing many anatomical papers on the larynx, spine, levator ani, phrenic nerve, and sacroiliac joint among others, all beautifully illustrated with lithographs from wood or copper engravings. The highlight of his scientific publications was his textbook of clinical anatomy published in three volumes between 1862 and 1867. In the second of these volumes, Luschka described slender bile ducts running along the gall bladder fossa, draining into the right hepatic or common hepatic duct.

Luschka's name is also associated with the two lateral foramina of the fourth ventricle through which cerebrospinal fluid enters the subarachnoid space (foramina

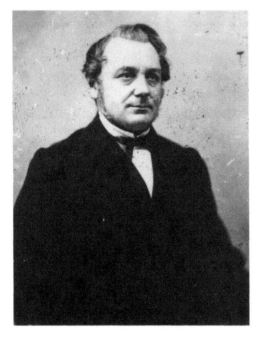

Portrait of Hubert Luschka. (By kind permission of the University of Tübingen Library [call number Dd 133f])

of Luschka) and small synovial joints between the lateral aspects of adjacent lower cervical vertebral bodies (uncovertebral joints).

Luschka gained a noble title and began using 'von' in his name in 1865. His first wife died after 13 years of marriage, leaving him with a young son and daughter. His second wife died unexpectedly after two years of marriage and he married a third time. He died in Tübingen.

References

Luschka H. *Die Anatomie des Menschen in Rücksicht auf die Bedürfnisse der praktischen Heilkunde bearbeitet.* Volumes I–III. Tübingen, 1862–1867.

Luschka H. *Die anatomie des menschlichen bauches.* Verlag der H Lauppschen, Buchhandlung, Tübingen, 1863, p.255.

Further reading

Dvorak J, Sandler A. Historical perspective. Hubert von Luschka. Pioneer of clinical anatomy. *Spine* 1994;**19**:2478–82.

McQuillanT, Manolas SG, Hayman JA, Kune GA. Surgical significance of the bile duct of Luschka. *Br J Surg* 1989;**76**:696–8.

Ko K, Kamiya J, Nagino M et al. A study of the subvesical bile duct (duct of Luschka) in resected liver specimens. *World J Surg* 2006;**30**:1316–20.

Sharif K, de Ville de Goyet J. Bile duct of Luschka leading to bile leak after cholecystectomy – revisiting the biliary anatomy. *J Pediatr Surg* 2003;**38**:E60.

Spanos CP, Syrakos T. Bile leaks from the duct of Luschka (subvesical duct): a review. *Langenbeck's Archives of Surgery* 2006;**391**:441–7.

Mayo Robson incision

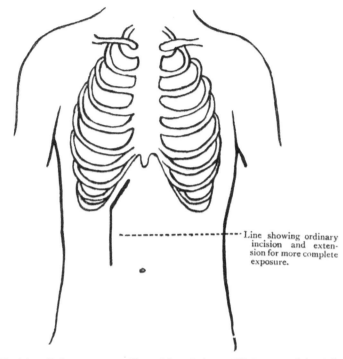

Line showing ordinary incision and extension for more complete exposure.

The Mayo Robson incision. (From Mayo Robson AW. *Diseases of the Gall-bladder and Bile-ducts, Including Gall-stones.* 3rd edition, Baillière, Tindall & Cox, London, 1904, Fig. 65, p.264)

The Mayo Robson incision is a right upper paramedian incision curved toward the xiphisternum designed to achieve optimum access for open biliary tract surgery. Mayo Robson said of the incision: "Whereas I used formerly to make a vertical incision through the linea semilunaris, I now always make my incision over the middle of the right rectus in a line parallel with its fibres, which are then separated by the finger, the posterior sheath of the rectus and peritoneum being divided together. Where the gall bladder is distended and there is no jaundice, a small incision of two or three inches only may be required; but when it is necessary to explore either the hepatic, common, or deeper part of the cystic duct, instead of prolonging the incision downwards, as was formerly done, I now carry it upwards in the interval between the ensiform cartilage [xiphisternum] and the right costal margin as high as possible, thus exposing the upper surface of the liver very freely" (Mayo Robson 1904). With the widespread application of laparoscopic techniques and curved 'rooftop' incisions, the incision is rarely used today.

131

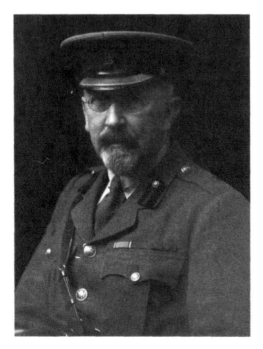

Sir Arthur William Mayo Robson by Walter Stoneman, 1917. (© National Portrait Gallery, London)

Arthur William Mayo Robson (1853–1933)

Mayo Robson was born in Filey, North Yorkshire, where his father, John Robson, was a chemist. He assumed the double-barreled surname in middle age (sometimes hyphenated as Mayo-Robson). He was an outstanding medical student in Leeds, winning most of the available prizes. After qualification, he was an anatomy demonstrator and then lecturer at the Leeds School of Medicine. In 1882, he became Assistant Surgeon at the General Infirmary at Leeds, progressing to Full Surgeon two years later, and then to Professor of Surgery at the Yorkshire College (the forerunner of Leeds University) in 1890, where he built his reputation for speed and skill. In 1902, he moved to London but never achieved quite the same surgical profile that he had enjoyed in Leeds. He was a Member of Council of the Royal College of Surgeons of England between 1893 and 1910 and Vice President twice. He was knighted in 1908.

Among his many fields of surgical interest, which included orthopaedics and gynaecology, he is best remembered for his expertise in biliary tract surgery. His classic text, *On Gall-stones and their Treatment*, was published in 1892, followed by *Diseases of the Gall-bladder and Bile-ducts* in 1897 and, with Percy Cammidge, *Gall-stones, Their Complications and Treatment* in 1909 (Mayo Robson 1892, 1897; Mayo Robson and Cammidge 1909). He also wrote books on surgery of the stomach and pancreas with his protegé, Berkeley Moynihan (1865–1936). His other eponymous legacies include Mayo Robson intestinal clamps and the Mayo Robson position on the operating table, a supine position with a thick wedge under the right flank and posterior ribs to push forward the spine and liver in operations on the gall bladder. In 1895 he was the first to report attempted surgical repair of a ruptured anterior cruciate ligament of the knee.

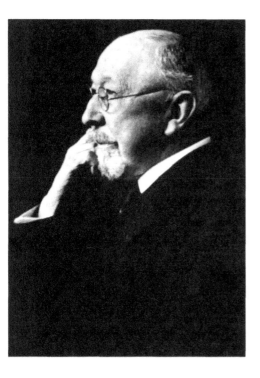

Sir Arthur Mayo Robson. (Reproduced with permission of the Leeds University Archive, UK)

During World War I, Mayo Robson served in the Army Medical Service in France, organising a hospital on the British lines, and then in Gallipoli and Egypt. For his military service he was made a Companion of the Royal Victorian Order in 1911 and a chevalier in the French Légion d'Honneur in 1921.

He was a short, sturdy man and although described as genial, he apparently came across at times as self-seeking. He was married twice and had three daughters. After retiring from surgical practice, he occasionally returned to Africa to hunt big game. During one of these expeditions, he was accidentally shot in both thighs by his carrier. When he died at the age of 80, he left numerous bequests to medical charities and to his alma mater, the Leeds General Infirmary.

References

Mayo Robson AW. *On Gall-stones and Their Treatment.* Cassell & Co., London, 1892.

Mayo Robson AW. *Diseases of the Gall-bladder and Bile-ducts, Including Gall-stones.* Baillière, Tindall & Cox, London,1897.

Mayo Robson AW, Cammidge P. *Gall-stones, Their Complications and Treatment.* Henry Frowde (Oxford University Press) 1909.

Further reading

D'A.P., W.R.L. Sir Arthur Mayo-Robson. *Ann R Coll Surg Engl* 1952;**11**:330–2.

Mayo Robson AW. *Diseases of the Gall-bladder and Bile-ducts, Including Gall-stones.* Baillière, Tindall & Cox, London, 3rd edition, 1904, pp249–64.

Mirizzi syndrome

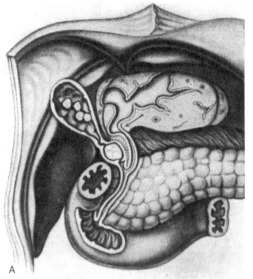
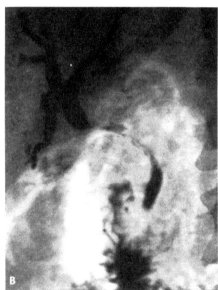

Schematic illustration (A) and operative cholangiogram (B) from Mirizzi's original description of common hepatic duct obstruction caused by a gallstone impacted in Hartmann's pouch or the cystic duct. (From Mirizzi PL. Sindrome del conducto hepatico. *Journal International de Chirurgie* 1948;**8**:731–77, Fig. 15, p.758 and Fig. 17, p.760)

Mirizzi described the condition now known as Mirizzi syndrome in an article published in 1948 (Mirizzi 1948). It is an uncommon cause of obstructive jaundice secondary to a gallstone impacted in Hartmann's pouch or the cystic duct causing obstruction of the common hepatic duct. Estimates suggest that Mirizzi's syndrome is encountered in 0.3–3% of cholecystectomies in adults. Mirizzi correctly surmised that the common hepatic duct obstruction was due to extrinsic pressure and local inflammation, although he erroneously implicated spasm of a circular muscle sphincter within the common hepatic duct as being important in the pathogenesis of the biliary obstruction.

Since the original description, Mirizzi's syndrome has been expanded and subdivided to include not only compression of the common hepatic duct but also the complication of cholecystobiliary fistula (to the common hepatic duct, common bile duct, or even the right hepatic duct).

Pablo Luis Mirizzi (1893–1964)

Born in Cordoba in Argentina to Italian immigrants, Mirizzi attended university in his native city and graduated in medicine in 1916. He subsequently studied clinical surgery at some of the best surgical centres in the United States, including the Mayo

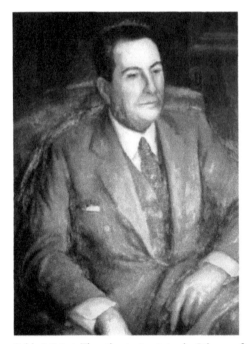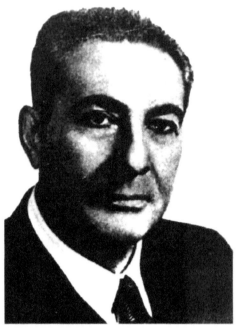

Pablo Mirizzi. The oil painting is in the Library of the Medical Sciences Faculty of the National School of Córdoba, Argentina. (Courtesy of Professor Jorge Cervantes, Professor of Surgery, National University of Mexico)

Clinic, and in Europe. He was appointed lecturer at the National University of Cordoba, Argentina in 1920 and Professor of Clinical Surgery in 1927.

Mirizzi focused on surgery of the abdomen, thorax and nervous system but is best remembered for his contributions to biliary tract surgery. In 1931, he performed the first ever intraoperative cholangiogram. His patient was a man named Edwviges Bustos de Jara, undergoing removal of common bile duct stones. Mirizzi published the technique in 1932 in an Argentinian surgical journal (Mirizzi 1932). Further articles in French and German followed but it was not until 1937 that he reported his experience of operative cholangiography in an American journal (Mirizzi 1937).

As a popular and skilled teacher, there was always competition for his surgical training courses. Mirizzi was a prolific writer, much of his output of more than 200 papers and numerous textbooks relating to biliary tract surgery. His contributions were recognised by honorary memberships and awards from around the world, especially from Europe and the Americas. In 1959, he became the first Latin American surgeon to become President of the International Congress of Surgery.

He had a deep affection for his native Cordoba and played an active role in the cultural life of the city, helping to develop the sport of fencing among other achievements. In 1968, a small square (plazoleta) in the city was named in his honour.

References

Mirizzi PL. La colangiografía durante las operaciones de las vías biliares. *Boletines y trabajos de la Sociedad de Cirugía de Buenos Aires* 1932;**16**:1133–61.

Mirizzi PL. Operative cholangiography. *Surg Gynecol Obstet* 1937;**65**:702–10.

Mirizzi PL. Sindrome del conducto hepatico. *Journal International de Chirurgie* 1948;**8**:731–77.

Further reading

Anon. Pablo Luis Mirizzi (1893–1964). *Bull Soc Int Chir* 1964;**23**:479–81.

Cervantes J, Rojas GA. Análisis de la práctica de la colangiografía transoperatoria en un periodo de veinte años [Analysis of the use of operative cholangiography in a 20-year period]. *Cirujano General* 2003;**25**:35–40.

Lai ECH, Lau WY. Mirizzi syndrome: history, present and future development. *ANZ J Surg* 2006;**76**:251–7.

Leopardi LN, Maddern GJ. Pablo Luis Mirizzi: the man behind the syndrome. *ANZ J Surg* 2007;**77**:1062–4.

Roake JA. Mirizzi syndrome: déjà vu again. *ANZ J Surg* 2007;**77**:1037.

Morison's pouch

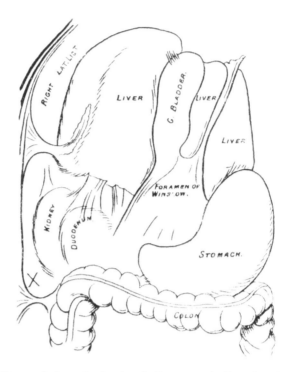

The pouch shown by drawing the liver upwards. X marks point for drainage. (From Morison R. The anatomy of the right hypochondrium relating especially to operations for gallstones. Br Med J 1894;2:968–71, Fig.1, p.968. Reproduced with permission of the BMJ Publishing Group)

Morison's pouch (hepatorenal pouch) is a peritoneal recess situated below the gall bladder and right lobe of the liver, anterior to the right kidney. First described in 1894, Morison advocated it as a useful site for providing efficient postoperative drainage, particularly following surgery for gallstones. The pouch has the following boundaries: anteriorly and superiorly the liver and gall bladder; posteriorly and inferiorly the mesocolon covering the kidney and duodenum; laterally the parietal peritoneum extending into the right paracolic gutter; and medially the posterior peritoneum over the spine, the epiploic foramen (of Winslow), and the free edge of the lesser omentum. Morison stated that the pouch had "natural barricades separating it from the general peritoneal cavity" and that it could be effectively drained by inserting a drain through the posterior parietal peritoneum immediately below the right kidney (X in the above figure). He noted that bile leaks and perforated duodenal ulcers led to fluid collections at this site, which is the most dependent part of the peritoneal cavity in the supine position.

James Rutherford Morison (1853–1939)

Morison was born at Hutton Henry, County Durham, where his father was a colliery doctor. At the age of 16 years, his father died from typhoid fever, which was endemic in many colliery villages at the time. This left Rutherford (he dropped the name 'James' in later years) to help support and educate his three brothers and two sisters. After graduating from Edinburgh University in 1876, he went straight into general practice in Hartlepool in the North of England. His interest in surgery flourished, nurtured by Lister, for whom he worked in Edinburgh ("the greatest man he had ever known"). He performed many operations in the homes of his patients. In 1878,

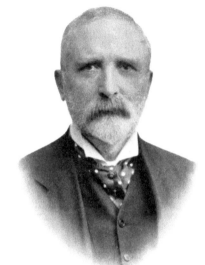

James Rutherford Morison.

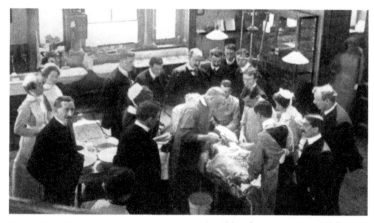

Rutherford Morison (centre) operating in the old Infirmary in 1906. (The Newcastle Medical Journal 1948;**23**:87–112)

he briefly visited Vienna, where he was inspired by Billroth. In 1881, in the face of considerable opposition, he was appointed as one of the two physicians to Hartlepool Hospital, where he performed most of the surgery carried out at the hospital.

In 1888, at the age of 35 years, Morison was persuaded to take up an appointment as Honorary Assistant Surgeon at the Royal Victoria Infirmary in Newcastle. A few years later, he visited Halsted at Johns Hopkins in Baltimore and was impressed by the latter's meticulous haemostasis. Morison became a full surgeon in Newcastle in 1897 and Professor of Surgery in 1910, before retiring in 1913. He was a staunch supporter of the British Medical Association and his political work improved the conditions of colliery doctors in the North of England. He was offered an honorary fellowship of the American College of Surgeons but this was never conferred since he considered that the journey to the USA would be too tiring.

Morison regarded teaching as his most important function and was popular, if somewhat dogmatic, with his students. He read medical journals every day. He worked hard and diligently but after his years in general practice avoided night work; any hour earlier than 10.00 a.m. he considered the middle of the night! His flair for diagnosis is illustrated by the following case: "A young girl, aged about 18, of great physical charms, for some months had complained of pain in her back, and she refused to walk because of this pain: no abnormal physical signs were ever detected: she had seen many physicians and surgeons, both in London and the provinces, who all made a diagnosis of neurosis [there being no radiology]. Whilst examining the case the patient unknowingly passed flatus, which Morison detected. He argued that no pretty girl would voluntarily do this during an examination. A diagnosis of tuberculous vertebra was made, and subsequent events confirmed the diagnosis" (Willan 1939).

His other surgical contributions included the use of an antiseptic paste (Bipp – a compound of bismuth, iodoform and paraffin) for treating contaminated wounds; transanal excision of intussuscepted distal colon cancer; and omentopexy for treating ascites complicating alcoholic cirrhosis (creating portosystemic collateral venous drainage). He prided himself on a meticulous operating technique comprisng strict antisepsis, catgut and silk sutures, moist gauze rolls with a 1-in porcelain ball attached by tape to avoid the complication of a retained swab, and marking the appropriate side of the patient with a large cross in all unilateral operations. He was capable of dismissing the scrub nurse on the spot for an error in the swab count.

Although married twice, he was a widower for many years. In general he enjoyed good health, which he attributed to daily exercise, walking or cycling to his consultations. After a major abdominal operation in 1923, he withdrew from his professional commitments to enjoy farming, golf, fishing, and curling. On his 80th birthday, 13 of his previous house surgeons presented him with an easy chair. Rutherford Morison is buried at St Boswells-on-Tweed in sight of the Eildon Hills that he loved.

M

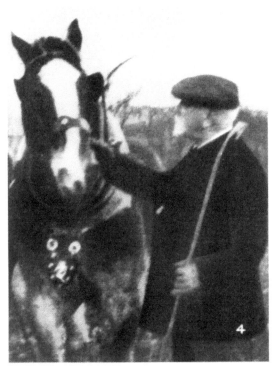

Morison at 77 years on his farm at St Boswells. (From the *Newcastle Medical Journal* 1948;**23**:87–112)

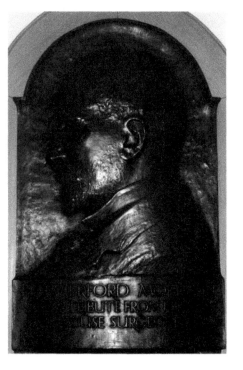

Life-size bronze plaque of Rutherford Morison (by Ernest Gillick, a London sculptor). Inscribed "Rutherford Morison, a tribute from his House Surgeons, 1888–1913". (Courtesy of the Royal Victoria Infirmary, Newcastle, England)

References

Grey Turner G. Rutherford Morison and his achievement. *The Newcastle Medical Journal* 1948;**23**:87–112.

Morison R. The anatomy of the right hypochondrium relating especially to operations for gallstones. *Br Med J* 1894;**2**:968–71.

Willan RJ. Obituary: Rutherford Morison. *Br Med J* 1939;**1**:139–42.

Further reading

Anon. Notes of Professor Rutherford Morison's clinic at Newcastle-upon-Tyne. *Br J Surg* 1913;**1**:686–94.

Dale G, Miller FWJ, Bramley K. Newcastle School of Medicine 1834–1984. *Sesquicentennial Celebrations Proceedings*. Faculty of Medicine, University of Newcastle upon Tyne, 1984.

Obituary of James Rutherford Morison. *Lancet* 1939;**1**:178–9.

Moynihan cholecystectomy forceps

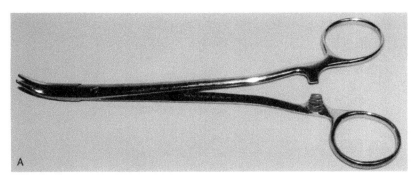

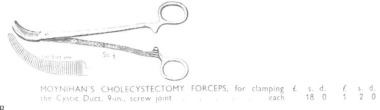

MOYNIHAN'S CHOLECYSTECTOMY FORCEPS, for clamping   £   s. d.   £   s. d.
the Cystic Duct, 9-in., screw joint   .   .   .   .   each   18   0   1   2   0

B

(A) Moynihan's cholecystectomy forceps made by Thackray (marked "THACKRAY ENGLAND STAINLESS STEEL"). This particular instrument was supplied to Thackray's works in Leeds as a 'model' example for further copies. (B) Taken from p. 66 of Chas F. Thackray Ltd. 1935 Catalogue of Surgical Instruments and Appliances, Surgical Sundries, Hospital Equipment and Sterilisation Apparatus. The price of 18 shillings was for nickel-plated forceps and one pound and two shillings for stainless steel forceps. The reference to "Sc ⅓" indicates that the instrument is depicted at one-third scale. (By permission of the Thackray Museum, Leeds, United Kingdom www.thackraymuseum.org)

In the past, surgeons would occasionally associate themselves with a particular instrument maker. This was the case with Berkeley Moynihan and Thackray. In 1902, Charles Frederick Thackray (1877–1934) and partner bought from Samuel Taylor a pharmacy he had established in Leeds. A few years later, they added a steriliser for dressings and from 1918 onwards began focussing on the production of surgical equipment. One of their main clients was Moynihan, Leeds' most prominent surgeon at that time. After Thackray's death his two sons continued the manufacturing business. In recent years, Thackray Instruments merged to become Seward Thackray, which still specialises in the production of surgical instruments.

Berkeley George Andrew Moynihan (1865–1936)

Moynihan was a British surgeon, born in Malta. His father was a distinguished military man who died when Berkeley was just 8 months old. As a young man Moynihan rejected a military career and chose to study medicine at Leeds Medical School, where 143

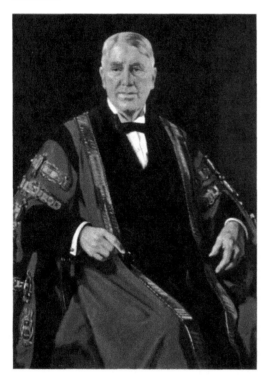

Sir Berkeley George Andrew Moynihan.*
Lord Moynihan of Leeds, President of
the Royal College of Surgeons of England
1926–1931. A painting by Richard Jack,
R.A. in 1927. (Courtesy of Leeds General
Infirmary)

he was taught by Arthur Mayo Robson (1853–1933). After graduating, he worked at
the Leeds Infirmary, becoming a full surgeon at the age of 41 years. Four years later,
in 1910, he was appointed to the Chair of Clinical Surgery. By this time, he had
already published two influential books, *Gall-stones and their Surgical Treatment* in
1904, and *Abdominal Operations* in 1905 (Moynihan 1904 and 1905).

During World War I, Moynihan served in France, rising to the rank of Major-
General. In 1917, he went on a lecture tour of the United States, where he spoke on
behalf of the British war effort. He gained many friends in America, to the extent
that he was invited to be the British Ambassador to Washington in 1929 (which he
declined).

Moynihan was an ardent supporter of Lister's antiseptic technique, stating that
"Every operation in surgery is an experiment in bacteriology" (Moynihan 1920).
He emphasised gentle tissue handling techniques rather than speed in surgery. His
dominant surgical interests were related to gallstones and gastric and duodenal ulcers,
although he also wrote on gunshot wounds and other surgical topics.

Moynihan received numerous honours from around the world. He was instrumental
in founding the *British Journal of Surgery* in 1913 and the Association of Surgeons of

Great Britain and Ireland in 1920. He was knighted in 1912, President of the Royal College of Surgeons of England between 1926 and 1931, and made a peer in 1929.

Moynihan was married with three children. He died of a cerebral haemorrhage just one week after his wife's death. At the time of his death, he was working on a Euthanasia Bill, which he planned to introduce to the House of Lords, in his capacity as Peer and as President of the Voluntary Euthanasia Legislation Society.

*Moynihan's image was also recorded in two busts and a bronze cast of his hands stands in the library at Leeds University Medical School.

References

Moynihan BGA. *Gall-stones and their Surgical Treatment*. WB Saunders & Co., Philadelphia, 1904.

Moynihan BGA. *Abdominal Operations*. WB Saunders & Co., Philadelphia, 1905.

Moynihan BGA. The ritual of a surgical operation. *Br J Surg* 1920;**8**:27–35.

Further reading

Bateman D. *Berkeley Moynihan – Surgeon*. Macmillan & Co., London, 1940.

Bunch G. Berkeley George Moynihan (1865–1963). Leeds Luminaries, Leeds University, 2001.

Plarr's Lives of the Fellows Online. The Royal College of Surgeons of England, 2006. http://livesonline.rcseng.ac.uk/biogs/E000226b.htm (Last accessed January 2009).

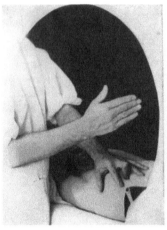
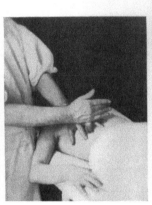
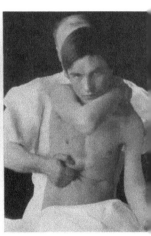

'Hammer-stroke percussion' and 'deep-grip palpation' to elicit Murphy's sign. (Reproduced with permission from *Five diagnostic methods of John B. Murphy. Surgical Clinics of John B. Murphy, M.D., at Mercy Hospital Chicago*. 1912;1:462, Figs 96–98 © Elsevier).

If Murphy's sign of acute cholecystitis is positive, gentle pressure in the right hypochondrium while the patient takes a deep inspiration is associated with a painful catch as the fundus of an inflamed gall bladder moves down and meets the pressure of the examiner's hand. The sign has a sensitivity and specificity of more than 90% in the diagnosis of acute cholecystitis but may be less reliable in the elderly (those older than 70 years of age).

According to Loyal Davis' biography, Murphy first presented this sign at an American Medical Association meeting around 1899 and was promptly accused by Frank Billings, a fellow surgeon in Chicago, of having stolen the observation from him. A description of the original technique of eliciting the sign, as demonstrated by Murphy, was published by a member of his staff in 1912 in the *Surgical Clinics of John B. Murphy, M.D., at Mercy Hospital Chicago* (Dowdall 1912). This entailed percussion of the right subcostal region immediately under the tip of the ninth costal cartilage at the height of inspiration after instructing the patient to take a deep breath; percussion was performed with the flexed middle finger of the left hand, using the right hand as a hammer to strike the dorsum of the left hand. Alternatively, 'deep-grip palpation' could be used to elicit the sign with the examiner's right hand curled up under the costal margin whilst the patient inspired deeply.

Murphy was a pioneer in a diverse range of surgical conditions including acute appendicitis (he performed the first appendicectomy in Chicago in 1889), thoracic surgery (artificial pneumothorax for pulmonary tuberculosis), arterial repair, intestinal anastomosis (for which he designed and promoted the Murphy button), fluid resuscitation (rectal saline infusion), and orthopaedics. He was a gifted clinical teacher and his *Surgical Clinics of John B Murphy, M.D., at Mercy Hospital, Chicago* later became the *Surgical Clinics of North America*. He was a founder of the American College of Surgeons and in 1911 was elected President of the American Medical Association. He received numerous awards including an honorary fellowship of the Royal College of Surgeons of England in 1913.

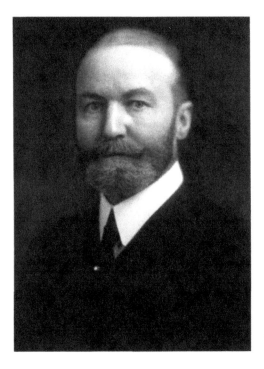

John B. Murphy. (Courtesy of the Chicago Surgical Society)

John Benjamin Murphy (1857–1916)

Born on a farm near Appleton, Wisconsin, to poor Catholic Irish émigrés, and christened John Murphy, he subsequently added the 'B' when, as a teenager, he noticed that most other boys at school had at least two initials. Murphy was heavily influenced by his local family doctor, who took him on as an assistant and tutored him with the help of a copy of *Gray's Anatomy*. Subsequently, Murphy studied medicine at Rush Medical College in Chicago, where he obtained his MD in 1880. After an internship at Cook County Hospital, he studied in Vienna with Billroth and with other European surgeons before returning to Chicago. Over the subsequent years he was Professor of Surgery at three medical schools: Rush Medical College; the College of Physicians and Surgeons (now the University of Illinois); and Northwestern University. For a while he was also Attending Surgeon at Cook County Hospital. In 1895 he became Chief of Surgery at Mercy Hospital, where his teaching became legendary and was acclaimed by such figures as William Mayo and Lord Berkeley Moynihan.

Murphy was a tall, powerful man with a short red beard and moustache and a high-pitched voice. At 27 years of age he married an 18-year-old former patient whom he had previously tended with typhoid fever. In 1887, their first child, a son, died from diphtheria at 6 weeks of age (despite Murphy performing a tracheotomy) and in the same year Murphy lost his sister and two brothers to tuberculosis. Family tragedy did not end there; he later lost one of his four daughters to complications of measles. His wife was a strong figure and, with her encouragement, Murphy acquired a large private practice in Chicago. He eventually became a millionaire and his wealth was a source of envy. He had a penchant for publicity, exemplified by his successful conservative treatment of Theodore Roosevelt's bullet wound of the chest in 1912. This, together with a tendency to criticise the practice of colleagues, made him unpopular with local surgeons, who claimed that his publications included only his successes. Murphy died of ischaemic heart disease at 59 years of age, after a long history of worsening angina. In his biography, Loyal Davis described him as having ambition, brilliance, strength and tenderness as well as egotism.

References

Davis L. *Surgeon Extraordinary: The Life of J. B. Murphy*. George G. Harrap, London, 1938.

Dowdall GD. Five diagnostic methods of John B. Murphy. *Surgical Clinics of John B. Murphy, M.D., at Mercy Hospital Chicago*. 1912,**1**:459–66.

Further reading

Adedeji OA, McAdam WA. Murphy's sign, acute cholecystitis and elderly people. *J R Coll Surg Edinb* 1996;**41**:88–9.

Beatty WK. J.B. Murphy, surgeon & teacher. *Proc Inst Med Chicago* 1979;**32**:102.

Ellis H. *Bailey and Bishop's Notable Names in Medicine and Surgery*. 4th edition. H.K.Lewis & Co.Ltd, London, 1983, pp174–8.

Griffith BH, Yao JST. A centennial history of the Chicago surgical society. *J Am Coll Surg* 2000;**191**:419–34.

Morgenstern L. J B Murphy, MD. Of buttons and blows. *Surg Endosc* 1998;**12**:359–60.

Musana K, Yale SH. John Benjamin Murphy (1857–1916). *Clin Med Res* 2005;**3**:110–112 (erratum 2005;**3**:132).

Schmitz RL, Oh TT. *The Remarkable Surgical Practice of John Benjamin Murphy*. University of Illinois Press, Urbana and Chicago, 1993.

Nardi provocation test

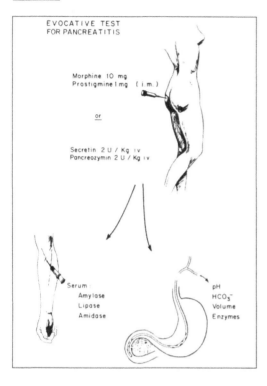

EVOCATIVE TEST
FOR PANCREATITIS

Morphine 10 mg
Prostigmine 1 mg   (i.m.)

or

Secretin 2 U / Kg iv
Pancreozymin 2 U / Kg iv

Serum
Amylase
Lipase
Amidase

pH
HCO₃⁻
Volume
Enzymes

Nardi test. The response of either serum enzymes or pancreatic secretion may be assayed. (From Nardi GL, Acosta JM. Papillitis as a cause of pancreatitis and abdominal pain: role of evocative test, operative pancreatography and histologic evaluation. *Ann Surg* 1966;**164**:611–18 , Fig. 1, p.612. © Lippincott, Williams & Wilkins)

The Nardi test, also known as the morphine-prostigmine provocation test, was originally reported as a method of diagnosing 'papillitis' or papillary stenosis in patients with recurrent pancreatitis of unknown aetiology. The aim was to predict patients who might benefit from sphincterotomy or sphincteroplasty. As described in 1966, the test involved the intramuscular injection of morphine (to induce sphincteric spasm) and prostigmine (to stimulate pancreatic exocrine secretion). If the patient's pain was reproduced and there was a fourfold increase in serum amylase or lipase, the test was positive. In retrospect, most of these patients had chronic pancreatitis.

The Nardi test is sometimes used today to detect sphincter of Oddi dysfunction in patients with apparent pancreatic or biliary pain but without evidence of an organic cause. However, it is of limited value because healthy volunteers can show similar rises in serum pancreatic enzyme concentrations and because more specific tests exist for diagnosing sphincter of Oddi dysfunction, such as cholecystokinin-HIDA scanning and biliary manometry.

George Lionel Nardi (1923–1989)

Nardi graduated in medicine from the University of Chicago in 1944. Except for a period working as a medical officer in the Navy, he spent his entire surgical career at Massachusetts General Hospital.

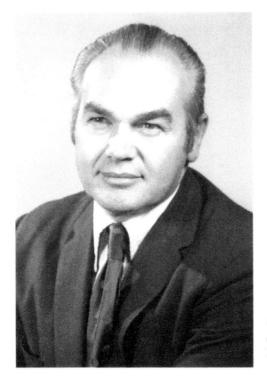

George L. Nardi. (Courtesy of the Department of Surgery, Massachusetts General Hospital, Boston, MA)

Nardi's clinical and laboratory research focused on pancreatitis and pancreatic cancer. In the 1950s, he discovered the link between primary hyperparathyroidism and pancreatitis. He died of cancer at the age of 66 years, leaving a wife and five children.

References

Nardi GL, Acosta JM. Papillitis as a cause of pancreatitis and abdominal pain: role of evocative test, operative pancreatography and histologic evaluation. *Ann Surg* 1966;**164**:611–8.

Further reading

Cope O, Culver PJ, Mixter CG Jr, Nardi GL. Pancreatitis, a diagnostic clue to hyperparathyroidism. *Ann Surg* 1957;**145**:857–63.

Lobo DN, Takhar AS, Thaper A, Dube MG, Rowlands BJ. The morphine-prostigmine provocation (Nardi) test for sphincter of Oddi dysfunction: results in healthy volunteers and in patients before and after transduodenal sphincteroplasty and transampullary septectomy. *Gut* 2007;**56**:1472–3.

Obituary. George L. Nardi, 66, Pancreas Illness Expert. *New York Times* December 6, 1989.

Ochsner trocar

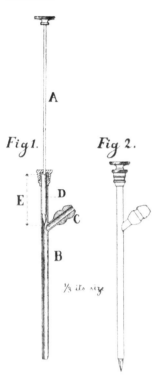

Fig1.

Fig 2.

A

E

D

C

B

⅓ its size

Edward Ochsner's combined trocar and aspirating device. A is a stylet, B the trocar tube, and C is attached to an aspirating syringe. (From Ochsner EH. An aspirating trocar. *Ann Surg* 1903;37:769–771, p.769.© Lippincott Williams & Wilkins)

Ochsner commissioned the construction of this steel trocar and aspirating device from a local instrument maker after experiencing dissatisfaction with other similar instruments. In his 1903 paper, he described the use of the trocar in more than 100 gall bladder operations, reporting that it was particularly useful in empyema.

Edward H. Ochsner (1868–1956)

Ochsner was an American surgeon who worked at the Augustana Hospital in Chicago from 1916. He graduated in medicine from Rush Medical College in 1894, and undertook postgraduate training in Vienna and Berlin. He was Professor of Clinical Surgery at the University of Illinois College of Physicians and Surgeons between 1900 and 1910, a charter member of the Chicago Surgical Society, and President of the Illinois State Charities Commission (1913–1917).

Edward is less well known than his younger brother, Albert J. Ochsner (1858–1925), and his cousin, Alton Ochsner (1896–1981), both of whom were famous surgeons. Albert was Professor of Surgery at the University of Illinois, founder and President of the American College of Surgeons, and best known for his work on the treatment of acute appendicitis. Alton was Professor of Surgery at Tulane University, New Orleans and a founder of the Ochsner Clinic Foundation.

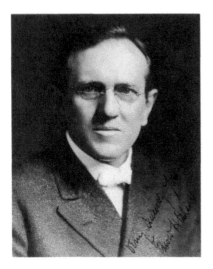

Edward H. Ochsner. (Courtesy of the Chicago History Museum, ICHi-59962)

Edward Ochsner's bibliography includes a wide range of surgical publications including those on liver cysts, congenital dislocation of the hip, the corpus luteum, and cervical exostoses. However, he also published books and articles on rehabilitation after illness and surgery, the benefits of colloidal gold in inoperable cancer, the US social security system, and medical education. In 1923, he wrote one of the earliest accounts of chronic fatigue syndrome (Ochsner 1923). His comments on medical matters were quoted widely. Of anaesthesia he stated: "We must learn that the giving of an anaesthetic is as important work as that of the chief surgical nurse, and almost, if not quite as important, as that of the operator himself."

References

Ochsner EH. An Aspirating Trocar. *Ann Surg* 1903;**37**:769–71.

Ochsner EH. *Chronic Fatigue Intoxication: a heretofore inadequately described affection*. GE Stechert & Co., New York, 1923.

Further reading

Council of the Chicago Medical Society. *Edward H Ochsner. History of Medicine and Surgery and Physicians and Surgeons of Chicago*. The Biographical Publishing Corporation; Chicago 1922, p.726.

Dr Ochsner, 88, noted Chicago surgeon, dies. *Chicago Daily Tribune* Jan 24, 1956.

Griffith BH, Yao JST. A centennial history of the Chicago surgical society. *J Am Coll Surg* 2000;**191**:419–34.

Ochsner, EH. *Physical Exercises for Invalids and Convalescents*. CV Mosby Co., St. Louis, Missouri, 1917.

Ochsner EH. The need for more well-trained practitioners of medicine. *Science* 1925;**62**:573–8.

Ochsner EH. *Social Security*. Social Security Press, Chicago, 1936.

Sphincter of Oddi

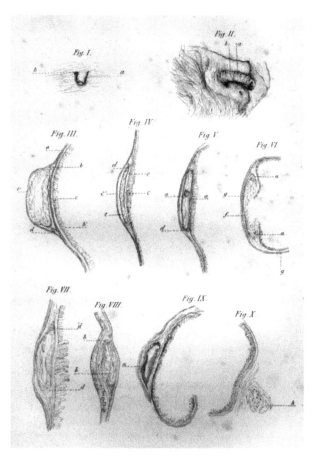

Oddi's drawings of the sphincter surrounding the distal common bile duct and pancreatic duct. I, dog; II, pig; III–VII, sheep and dog; VIII, man; IX, birds (domestic pigeon, common hen, and hen pheasant). (From Oddi R. Di una speciale disposizione a sfintere allo sbocco del coledoco. *Annali della Libera Università di Perugia* 1886–1887;**II**:249–65, Table IX, p.265. By kind permission of the Biblioteca di Medicina, University of Perugia, Italy)

The sphincter of Oddi refers to the smooth muscle that surrounds the termination of the common bile duct and pancreatic duct. Francis Glisson had described the circular muscle fibres of the sphincter over 200 years earlier in *Anatomia hepatis* (1654). Oddi acknowledged this but regarded Glisson's comments as a hypothesis rather than based on detailed observations. Furthermore, Glisson believed that the primary function of the 'sphincter' was to prevent chyle entering the bile duct, rather than to regulate the flow of bile into the duodenum. The sphincter had also been described in the cat by Simon Gage in 1879 in the first issue of the *American Quarterly Microscopy Journal* (Gage 1879).

Oddi's histological studies confirmed the sphincter in a wide variety of animals including humans, established that it was distinct from the smooth muscle of the duodenal wall, and described the part of the sphincter surrounding the pancreatic duct. He was the first to measure the resistance of the sphincter and his studies led him to conclude that the sphincter controlled the intermittent flow of bile from the liver to the duodenum. He also suggested that dysfunction of the sphincter might

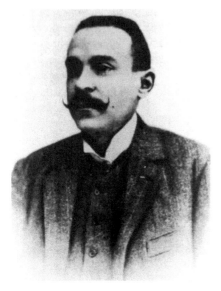

Ruggero Oddi (in 1906). (Courtesy of the National Library of Medicine)

explain some biliary tract pathology and transient forms of obstructive jaundice, a prediction manifest today in sphincter of Oddi dysfunction and biliary dyskinesia. After his move to Genoa, Oddi continued to study the sphincter, focusing on its autonomic innervation, leading to a summary monograph in 1897 entitled *The Physiopathology of the Biliary Tree* (cited in Morelli and Sorcetti 1988).

Ruggero Ferdinando Antonio Giuseppe Vincenzo Oddi (1864–1913)

Oddi was born in Perugia, Italy where his father was an archivist at the local hospital. He began his medical studies at the University of Perugia where, as a 23-year-old fourth-year student, he conducted his famous research into the anatomy and physiology of the sphincter at the termination of the common bile duct. Since the University of Perugia could not at that time award a medical degree, Oddi transferred to the University of Bologna, where he extended his studies on the sphincter. In 1889 he gained his degree in medicine and surgery, subsequently moving to the Institute of Physiology in Florence and later to Strasburg.

Oddi was appointed Director of the Physiology Institute at the University of Genoa in 1894 at just 29 years of age. Here, his research focused on the physiology of the nervous system, respiratory metabolism, and pregnancy. He achieved substantial academic recognition in Italy during his seven years in this position. Then, for reasons probably related to events in his family, illness, drug addiction, and/or fiscal impropriety, Oddi's career went into freefall, causing him to be removed from his position and leave Italy.

In 1891, Oddi married 23-year-old Teresa Bresciani Bartoli a few months after their first child was born; the couple had a second child in 1893. Little is known about the fate of his family but their disappearance in 1901 from registers in both Florence and Perugia suggests serious family problems. In Genoa, Oddi had become friends with an influential aristocrat, Stefano Capranica, who owned the physiology laboratory that Oddi used for his research. After the death of his mistress, Capranica became addicted to morphine and experienced a spiritual crisis, both of which appeared to have a profound effect on Oddi. Prior to his death in 1899, Capranica donated all his property to the Genovese Curia, which duly confiscated Oddi's laboratory, uncovering serious financial irregularities and Oddi's probable drug abuse in the process. Oddi either resigned or was relieved of his position in the scandal that followed.

In parallel with these events, Oddi had undergone surgery for appendicitis in 1898 and, two years later, for bowel obstruction. To escape the turmoil, he moved to Brussels (where he was treated for depression) and thence to the Belgian Congo, where he worked as a doctor. However, ill health, mental instability, and possibly ongoing narcotic abuse forced him to return to Belgium six months later. In 1905, he returned to Perugia, where he practiced medicine, widely advocating the administration of Vitaline (a compound of glycerin, sodium borate, ammonium chloride and alcohol) for infectious and malignant diseases. After the death of one of his patients, he was accused of manslaughter and charged with "abusive commerce of medicinal products". He became a broken man and left Perugia for Tunisia in 1911, where he died two years later at the age of 48 years.

References

Gage S. The ampulla of Vater and the pancreatic ducts in the domestic cat. *Am Quart Micro J* 1879;**1**:1–20.

Glisson F. *Anatomia Hepatis*. Du-Gardianis, Impensis Octaviani Pullein, Londoni, 1654.

Morelli A, Sorcetti F. Ruggero Oddi's life. *Zeitschrift fur Gastroenterologie Verhhandlungsband* 1988;**23**:203–7.

Oddi R. Di una speciale disposizione a sfintere allo sbocco del coledoco. *Annali della Libera Università di Perugia* 1886–1887;**II**:249–65.

Further reading

Belloni L. Über Leben und Werk von Ruggero Oddi (1864–1913), dem Entdecker des Schliessmuskels des Hauptgallenganges. *Medizinhistorische Journal* 1966;**1**:96–109.

Howard JM, Hess W. *History of the Pancreas: Mysteries of a Hidden Organ*. Springer, Heidelberg, 2002.

Kanne JP, Rohrmann CA, Lichtenstein JE. Eponyms in radiology of the digestive tract: historical perspectives and imaging appearances. Part 2. Liver, biliary system, pancreas, peritoneum, and systemic disease. *Radiograhics* 2006;**26**:465–80.

Sphincter of Oddi

Loukas M, Spentzouris G, Tubbs RS, Kapos T, Curry B. Ruggero Ferdinando Antonio Guiseppe Vencenzo Oddi. *World J Surg* 2007; **31**:2260–2265.

Modlin IM, Ahlman H. Oddi: the paradox of the man and the sphincter. *Arch Surg* 1994;**129**:549–56.

Oddi R. D'une disposition à sphincter spéciale de l'ouverture du canal cholédoque (1). *Archives Italiennes de Biologie* 1887;**8**:317–22.

Oddi R. Sulla tonicita dello sfintere del coledocho. *Archivio Per Le Scienze Mediche* 1888;**12**:333–9.

Trancanelli V. Ruggero Oddi and the discovery of the common bile duct sphincter. *Minerva Medica* 1993;**84**:57–66.

NOTES ON THE ARREST OF HEPATIC HEMOR-
RHAGE DUE TO TRAUMA.

BY J. HOGARTH PRINGLE, F.R.C.S.,

OF GLASGOW,

Lecturer on Surgery in Queen Margaret College, Surgeon to the Glasgow Royal Infirmary.

Title of Pringle's 1908 article. (From Pringle JH. Notes on the arrest of hepatic hemorrhage due to trauma *Ann Surg* 1908;**48**:541–9)

In 1908, Pringle reported an 11-year experience of managing bleeding from the injured liver after blunt liver trauma. None of his eight reported cases survived: three died from multiple injuries soon after admission to hospital, one refused operation and died three days later, and the other four died despite laparotomy and attempts to control the haemorrhage. After the death of the first patient, Pringle conceived the idea of temporary inflow occlusion. Thus, in the second operative case, Pringle instructed his assistant to compress the portal vein and hepatic artery between a finger and thumb in the anterior boundary of the epiploic foramen (of Winslow). This manoeuvre "…completely arrested all bleeding…". He then packed the depths of the torn hepatic parenchyma and sutured the margins but unfortunately the patient died soon after the operation.

Following these clinical observations, Pringle decided to investigate the effects of temporary hepatic inflow occlusion in experimental animals. He carried out these studies in the Pathological Institute in Vienna. He occluded the portal triad for up to one hour in four rabbits, during which he successfully performed hepatic lobectomy. He concluded that his manoeuvre was probably safe to use in humans. Pringle used the technique in his third and fourth operative cases of blunt liver trauma and although both patients died the fourth patient's bleeding was successfully controlled by temporary inflow occlusion and perihepatic packing; unfortunately, this man died four days later from pulmonary complications.

Whilst blunt liver injury is now frequently managed non-operatively, persistent haemorrhage is an indication for surgery. Pringle's manoeuvre is useful in the temporary control of haemorrhage. It is also employed during hepatic resection to minimise blood loss. The adult human liver comfortably tolerates one hour of inflow occlusion but longer periods are possible if the Pringle manoeuvre is applied intermittently or after ischaemic preconditioning.

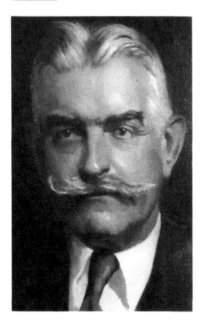

Portrait of James Hogarth Pringle by William Dring, R.A.
(Reproduced by kind permission of the President and
Council of the Royal College of Physicians and Surgeons
of Glasgow)

James Hogarth Pringle (1863–1941)

Pringle was Australian by birth. He was born in Parramatta, New South Wales,
Australia. His father, George Hogarth Pringle, was a well-known surgeon in Sydney
and a friend of Joseph Lister. Pringle's ancestors included William Hogarth, the
famous British artist and satirist, and Charles Dickens' sister. Pringle graduated
from Edinburgh University in 1885 and, after a period of study in Europe, he was
appointed to the staff at Glasgow Royal Infirmary, becoming Senior Surgeon in
1890.

His life centred around the hospital, being responsible for most of the routine and
emergency surgery. He made several major contributions to trauma, orthopaedics
and vascular surgery. He was the first surgeon in Britain to perform hindquarter
amputation; he described the use of a reversed autologous saphenous vein graft
to repair the injured brachial artery and to replace a popliteal aneurysm; and he
experimented with xenotransplantation, using urethral tissue from a bullock to repair
a male urethral stricture. Pringle kept detailed notes and was an advocate of long-
term follow up of patients; he recorded the outcome of his patients with cutaneous
melanoma up to 38 years later.

Pringle championed the role of nursing staff and women in medicine. With his
encouragement, the first nurse training school in Britain was established. He was the
first lecturer in surgery and demonstrator in anatomy to Glasgow's Queen Margaret
College for Women medical students founded in 1899. He could be rather abrupt
and forbidding but was said to be kind hearted by those who knew him well. He

took obligatory retirement from his position as Senior Surgeon at Glasgow Royal Infirmary at 60 years of age but he continued to teach surgical trainees and medical students for many years thereafter.

References

Pringle JH. Notes on the arrest of hepatic hemorrhage due to trauma. *Ann Surg* 1908;**48**:541–9.

Further reading

Grey Turner G. Obituary. James Hogarth Pringle. *Br Med J* 1941;**1**:734.

Gurey LE, Swan KG, Swan KG. James Hogarth Pringle. *Journal of Trauma Injury, Infection, and Critical Care* 2005;**58**:201–5.

Miln DC. James Hogarth Pringle, 1863–1941. *Br J Surg* 1964;**51**:241–5.

Obituary. James Hogarth Pringle MB FRCS, Glasgow. *Glasgow Medical Journal* 1941;**135**:153–7.

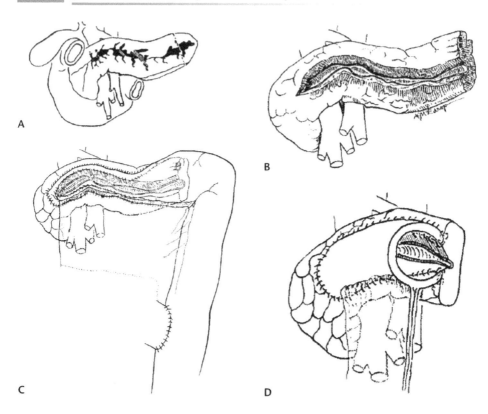

(A) Appearance of pancreatic ducts, as seen in some pancreatograms. Note the alternate dilatations and stenoses that are commonly present. (B) Pancreatic duct split open. Catarrhal inflammation is frequently found at the stenotic narrowing, and calcification may be present at these spots. (C) Pancreaticojejunostomy with opened pancreas and opened jejunum, so that the pancreaticojejunostomy is a side-to-side anastomosis. Note the anterior position of the jejunal mesentery. (D) Cross-section of the pancreaticojejunal anastomosis. (Reproduced from Puestow CB and Gillesby WJ. Retrograde surgical drainage of pancreas for chronic relapsing pancreatitis. *AMA Archives of Surgery* 1958;**76**:899 Fig. 1 & 902 Fig. 2, with permission of the American Medical Association)

The Puestow procedure or longitudinal pancreaticojejunostomy involves making a longitudinal incision in the pancreatic duct and anastomosing it to a segment of jejunum. In their paper published in 1958, Puestow and Gillesby acknowledged that both pancreatic duct drainage via a sphincteroplasty and caudal pancreatico-jejunostomy (after resection for pancreatic carcinoma) had been reported previously (Puestow and Gillesby 1958). Their contribution was to suggest extended pancreatic drainage via an incision along the length of the duct, opening any pancreatic duct strictures and internally draining the duct into the jejunum. They considered that this procedure relieved pain from pancreatic ductal obstruction and, that by relieving obstruction and preserving parenchyma, some pancreatic regeneration was possible, leading to improved exocrine function.

In their original description, Puestow and Gillesby removed the spleen and amputated the tail of the pancreas to access the distal pancreatic duct, which was then split open proximally "as far to the right as is possible". A Roux-en-Y pancreaticojejunostomy was fashioned in two layers using one of several techniques. In the first, the opened pancreas was inserted into the open end of a limb of jejunum, which was then sutured circumferentially around the neck of the pancreas. In the second, the standard side-to-side longitudinal pancreaticojejunostomy was performed, invaginating only the tip of the amputated pancreatic tail and suturing the jejunum as an anterior onlay graft to the cut edge of the pancreatic parenchyma. Yet a third anastomotic technique, pancreaticogastrostomy, was also described in two patients. In all cases, the abdomen was closed with drainage.

Puestow began performing the procedure early in 1953 and reported his experience of 21 patients with Gillesby in 1958. Most of his patients had alcohol-induced chronic pancreatitis. There were no surgical deaths and patients were relieved of pain.

Two years later, Partington and Rochelle (1960) reported a modification of the Puestow procedure. They preserved the spleen and pancreatic tail, locating and opening the pancreatic duct from the anterior surface of the gland rather than by amputating its tail. Other authors subsequently recommended a mucosa-to-mucosa anastomosis rather than the jejunal mucosa to cut edge of pancreatic parenchyma described by Puestow and Gillesby.

Charles Bernard Puestow (1902–1972)

Charles Puestow was born in the USA and studied medicine at the University of Pennsylvania, gaining an MS and PhD from the University of Minnesota. He had a distinguished career in World War II as Commanding Officer of the 27th Evacuation Hospital, receiving numerous medals including the Croix de Guerre with Palm. After returning to civilian life he became Chief of Surgery at the University of Illinois College of Medicine.

In 1957, whilst working at the Hines Memorial Veterans Hospital in Illinois and as President of the Chicago Surgical Society, Puestow and his colleague, William Gillesby, proposed a treatment for chronic pancreatitis, which became known as the Puestow procedure. His paper, published in 1958, was entitled *Retrograde surgical drainage of pancreas for chronic relapsing pancreatitis*.

Puestow published two books *Emergency Care, Surgical and Medical* along with Warren H Cole (1898–1990) and *Surgery of the Biliary Tract, Pancreas and Spleen* (1953), the latter going to four editions (Cole and Puestow 1951; Puestow 1953).

Puestow procedure (longitudinal pancreaticojejunostomy)

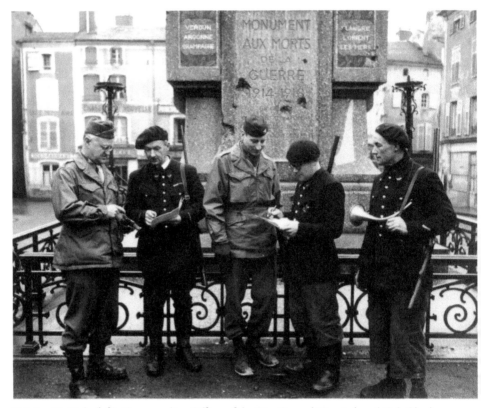

Col. Lee D. Cady (left), Commanding Officer of the 21st General Hospital, and Col. Charles Puestow (centre), Commanding Officer of the 27th Evacuation Hospital, meet with French foresters after an unsuccessful wild boar hunt on March 8, 1945. The subjects are standing in front of Le Monument aux Morts de la Grande Guerre in Mirecourt, France. (Reproduced by permission of the Becker Medical Library, Washington University School of Medicine)

References

Cole WH, Puestow CB. *Emergency Care: Surgical and Medical.* Appleton Century Crofts, 1951.

Partington PF, Rochelle REL. Modified Puestow procedure for retrograde drainage of the pancreatic duct. *Ann Surg* 1960;**152**:1037–43.

Puestow CB. *Surgery of the Biliary Tract, Pancreas & Spleen.* Year Book Publishers, Chicago, 1953.

Puestow CB, Gillesby WJ. Retrograde surgical drainage of pancreas for chronic relapsing pancreatitis. *Arch Surg* 1958;**76**:898–907.

Further reading

Griffith BH, Yao JST. A centennial history of the Chicago Surgical Society. *J Am Coll Surg* 2000;**191**:419–34.

R Ranson's criteria

On admission:
  Age > 55 years
  WBC > 16,000/μl
  Blood glucose > 200 mg%
  SLDH > 700 IU%
  SGOT > 250 S-F.U%

During initial 48 hours:
  Hematocrit decrease > 10%
  BUN rise > 5 mg%
  Serum calcium < 8 mg%
  Arterial PO_2 < 60 mm Hg
  Base deficit > 4 mEq/l
  Estimated fluid sequestration > 6 L

Eleven early grave prognostic signs apparent within 48 hours of diagnosis as identified by Ranson. (From Ranson JH, Rifkind KM, Roses DF, Fink SD, Eng K, Localio SA. Objective early identification of severe acute pancreatitis. *Am J Gastroenterol* 1974;**61**:446)

Ranson made a major contribution to the understanding and treatment of acute pancreatitis, publishing numerous clinical and experimental studies in this field. In 1974, he and his colleagues published a prognostic scoring system, which came to be known as Ranson's criteria or Ranson's Prognostic Score used to determine the severity of acute pancreatitis and predict mortality. In this paper, he analysed clinical and laboratory features from 100 patients with acute pancreatitis, 74 of whom had disease secondary to alcohol and 14 with biliary tract related pancreatitis. Patients were divided into those who required intensive care or died and those with milder disease. Eleven predictive criteria were identified: 62% of patients with more than three criteria within 48 hours of admission died and a further 33% were seriously ill compared with 3% and 11%, respectively of those with fewer than three criteria. Although serum amylase was elevated in all patients during the course of their disease, it was normal in five cases on admission and did not emerge as an independent prognostic marker. Signs on plain radiographs were also analysed but proved to be too variable to be of prognostic value.

Ranson's criteria assisted in the triage of patients with acute pancreatitis and assessment of their quality of care. By allowing comparison of stratified groups of patients, the scoring system became a cornerstone of therapeutic studies in acute pancreatitis for more than two decades. In a modified version of the scheme known as the Glasgow (Imrie) score, the number of criteria was reduced from 11 to eight or nine (Blamey et al 1984). Other prognostic scoring systems based on physiological parameters (e.g. Acute Physiology and Chronic Health Evaluation, APACHE II, and the Early Warning Score) (Garcea et al 2006), serum inflammatory markers (e.g. C-reactive protein concentration), or radiological findings (e.g. CT grading scores of the extent of pancreatic necrosis) were subsequently developed, some of which offered greater versatility in monitoring the progress of individual patients with acute pancreatitis.

Ranson's criteria

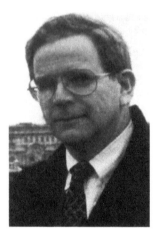

John H.C. Ranson. (Kindly provided by Professor H. Leon Pachter, Department of Surgery, NYU School of Medicine)

John H.C. Ranson (1938–1995)

Ranson was born in Bangalore, India, where his English father was a missionary. The family moved to New York when he was nine years old and John was sent to boarding school in Massachusetts. He returned to England to study medicine at Oxford University, graduating in 1963. After postgraduate training at St Bartholomew's Hospital in London and Bellevue Hospital in New York, he joined the faculty of New York University Medical Center, where he later became Professor and Chief of Surgery. Throughout his career he remained interested in pancreatic disorders and was a founding Associate Editor of the journal *Pancreas*.

Ranson was honoured by many prestigious medical societies including the New York State Medical Society and the Danish Medical Society. At the time of his death, he was President of the Society of Surgery of the Alimentary Tract. By close associates, he was described as a religious and principled individual, devoted to his wife and two children. He died of multiple myeloma at 57 years of age.

References

Blamey SL, Imrie CW, O'Neill J, Gilmour WH, Carter DC. Prognostic factors in acute pancreatitis. *Gut* 1984;**25**:1340–6.

Garcea G, Jackson B, Pattenden CJ, Sutton CD, Neal CP, Dennison AR, Berry DP. Early warning scores predict outcome in acute pancreatitis. *J Gastrointest Surg* 2006;**10**:1008–15.

Ranson JHC, Rifkind KM, Roses DF, Fink SD, Eng K, Localio SA. Objective early identification of severe acute pancreatitis. *Am J Gastroenterol* 1974;**61**:443–51.

Further reading

Frey CF. Commitment and fulfillment: The life of John H.C. Ranson. *J Gastrointest Surg* 1997;**1**:92–6.

Reber HA. Obituary. John H.C. Ranson, MD. *Pancreas* 1996;**12**:215.

Retzius' veins

The veins of Retzius are retroperitoneal portocaval anastomoses. They connect portomesenteric venous tributaries around the duodenum and colon with tributaries of the inferior vena cava. Retzius discovered these venous connections after ligating the distal portal vein in fresh cadavers and forcibly injecting the proximal segment with coloured dyes. He identified a plexus of small veins in the retroperitoneum that connected portomesenteric veins around the duodenum and colon with the inferior vena cava and renal veins. Unfortunately, his report contained no illustrations.

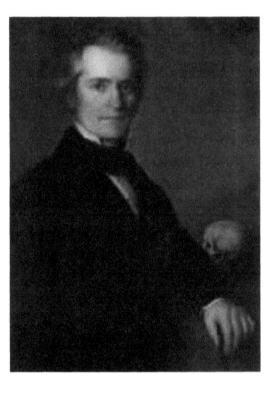

Anders Retzius. Painted in 1854 by Gustaf Uno Troilii. The picture now hangs in the Faculty Club *Svarta räfven* [The Black Fox] at the Karolinska Institutet. (© Karolinska Institutet)

Anders Adolf Retzius (1796–1860)

Retzius was a Swedish anatomist and anthropologist whose name is associated with numerous anatomical features including Retzius' gyri in the brain and the retropubic space of Retzius (also called the cave of Retzius). His father was a distinguished professor of natural history in Lund. Retzius completed his medical studies at the University of Lund in 1819, gaining his medical doctorate a year later with a dissertation on the anatomy of cartilaginous fishes. After working at the Stockholm Veterinary Institute, he was appointed Professor of Anatomy at the Karolinska Medico-Kirurgiska Institutet at just 28 years of age. Here, his work centred on comparative and clinical anatomy as well as anthropology. He was particularly

165

interested in the structure of teeth and ethnic variation in cranial morphology. The latter studies led him to express controversial racial opinions, which to some extent tarnish his modern day reputation.

Further reading

Anders Adolf Retzius. http://www.whonamedit.com/doctor.cfm/3292.html © 1994–2009 Ole Daniel Enersen. (Last accessed January 2009).

Ibukuro K, Tsukiyama T, Mori K, Inoue Y. Veins of Retzius at CT during arterial portography: anatomy and clinical importance. *Radiology* 1998;**209**:793–800.

Larsell O. Anders Adolf Retzius (1796–1860). *Ann Med Hist* 1924;**6**:16–24.

Retzius A. Bemerkungen über Anastomosen zwischen der Pfortader und der unteren Hohlader ausserhalb der Leber. *Zeitschrift für Physiologie* 1835;**5**:105–6.

Beiträge zur Morphologie der Säugerleber.

Von

Dr. Hugo Rex,

Prosektor am deutschen anatomischen Institut in Prag.

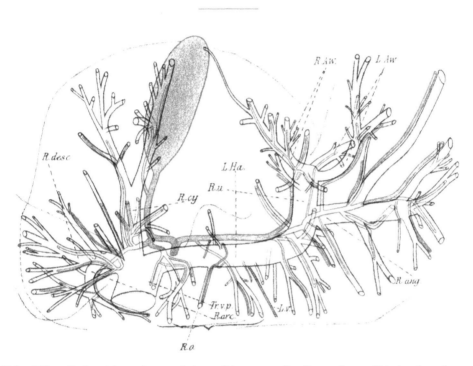

Title of Hugo Rex's article on the morphology of the mammalian liver and one of his sketches of the branches of the portal vein and hepatic artery. (From Rex H. Beiträge zur Morphologie der Säugerleber. *Morphologisches Jahrbuch* 1888;14:517–617)

In his 1888 article on the morphology of the mammalian liver, Rex described the branching of the portal vein. He commented that the left portal vein has a sagittally running segment which, at its ventral end, is attached to the ligamentum teres. Rex called the slight expansion of the portal vein at this point and this part of the liver, the 'umbilical recess', emphasising that it represented an important border zone within the left lobe of the liver.

In recent years, the Rex umbilical recess has been used as an important anatomical landmark in an operation to correct extrahepatic portal hypertension from congenital

167

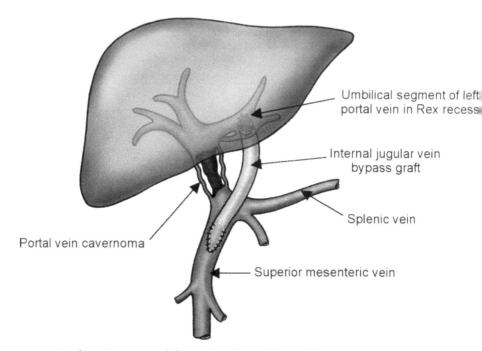

Umbilical segment of left
portal vein in Rex recess

Internal jugular vein
bypass graft

Splenic vein

Superior mesenteric vein

Portal vein cavernoma

Rex shunt (mesenterico-left portal vein bypass) for extrahepatic portal hypertension.

or acquired portal vein occlusion. In the standard Rex shunt operation, which is also known as the mesenterico-left portal bypass procedure, a vascular graft is inserted between the superior mesenteric vein and the umbilical segment of the left portal vein within the Rex recess of the liver. In contrast to portosystemic shunts, the Rex shunt restores hepatopetal portal flow, thus achieving near-normal hepatic circulatory physiology.

Hugo Rex (1861–1936)

Rex was born in Prague into a medical family. His father was a military doctor in the Czech territory of Bohemia, then part of the Austro-Hungarian empire. Rex gained his medical degree from the German University in Prague in 1885, where he remained to continue with his anatomical studies. He travelled to Nepal, Norway and Paris to collect material for his thesis, which focused on the comparative anatomy of the liver and which he completed in 1889. Unfortunately, his skilled preparations of the hepatic vasculature relied on paraffin injections and these have not survived to this day.

Rex was appointed Professor of Comparative Anatomy at the German University in Prague and occupied this post until his retirement in 1931. He also published reports

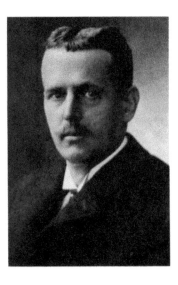

Portrait photograph of Hugo Rex. (Courtesy of Professor Oldrich Eliska, Institute of Anatomy, Charles University, Prague)

on the anatomy of the cerebral veins in cartilaginous fishes and amphibians and the muscles of the jaw and eyes in birds. He personally collected many of his specimens, even wading into fishponds to acquire seagull eggs. His biological preparations and reconstructions were widely acclaimed. Described as a quiet, introverted and modest man he was held in high regard by his students and colleagues.

References

Rex H. Beiträge zur Morphologie der Säugerleber. *Morphologisches Jahrbuch* 1888;**14**:517–617.

Further reading

Chen VT, Wei J, Liu YC. A new procedure for management of extrahepatic portal obstruction. *Arch Surg* 1992;**127**:1358–60.

de Ville de Goyet J, Clapuyt P, Otte JB. Extrahilar mesenterico-left portal shunt to relieve extrahepatic portal hypertension after partial liver transplant. *Transplantation* 1992;**53**:231–2.

de Ville de Goyet J, Alberti D, Clapuyt P, et al. Direct bypassing of extrahepatic portal venous obstruction in children: a new technique for combined hepatic portal revascularization and treatment of extrahepatic portal hypertension. *J Pediatr Surg* 1998;**33**:597–601.

Großer O. Obituary of Hugo Rex. In: *Bericht. Über das Studienjahr 1935/36 der Deutschen Universität in Prag Erstattet von Prorektor Prof. Dr. Karl Hilgenreiner. Nachrufe. Zur Altersfrage der Erdrinde von Prof. Dr. Michael Stark Rektor 1936/37.* Selbstverlag der Deutschen Universität, Prag, 1937, pp53–4.

Hlaváčková L, Svobodný P. *Biographisches Lexikon der Deutschen Medizinischen Fakultät in Prag 1883–1945.* Deutschen Universität, Prag.

Riedel's lobe

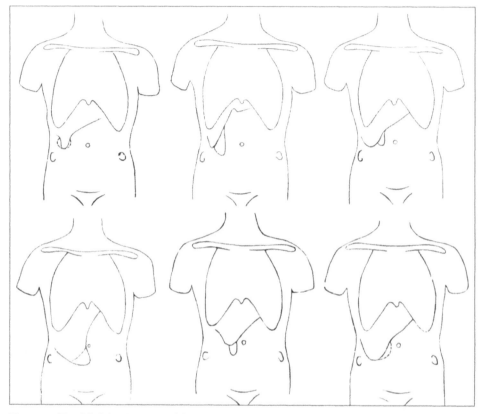

Varieties of Riedel's lobe. (From Riedel B. Ueber den zungenförmigen Fortsatz des rechten Leberlappens und seine pathognostische Bedeutung für die Erkrankung der Gallenblase nebst Bemerkungen über Gallensteinoperationen. *Berliner Klinische Wochenschrift* 1888;29:577–81)

In 1888, Riedel described a tongue-like inferior projection from the inferior border of the right lobe of the liver superficial to or to the right of the gall bladder. He reported this finding in seven women, aged between 30 and 49 years, six of whom had cholecystitis. Each had a palpable mass in the right hypochondrium, which was confirmed as liver tissue at surgery or at postmortem. Because of the association with chronic cholecystitis and, in some cases, apparent resolution of the clinical finding after surgery, Riedel postulated that perihepatic inflammation with adhesions could cause the deformity by traction. He also suggested that it might arise from wearing tight corsets.

Since the original description, there has been controversy about whether Riedel's lobe is congenital or acquired, its overall frequency, and whether it is more commonly found in women. In an analysis of 2604 Tc-99m sulfur colloid liver scintigrams, Sham et al (1978) found evidence of a Riedel's lobe in 4.5% of women and 2.1% of men. If Riedel's lobe is defined as being present when the liver extends caudal to the most inferior part of the costal margin, it appears to be a common finding in both men and women (Gillard et al 1998). Rarely, the enlargement is pedunculated (James et al 1963).

Bernhard Moritz Carl Ludwig Riedel (1846–1916)

Born in Mecklenburg, a federal state of former East Germany, Riedel graduated in medicine from the University of Rostock in 1872 and, for the next three years, was prosector at the Institute of Anatomy in Rostock, working under the anatomist

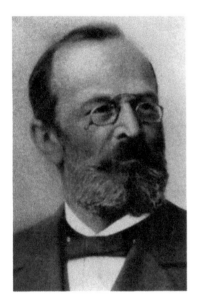

Bernhard Riedel. (From Biographisches Lexikon der hervorragenden Ärzte der letzten fünfzig Jahre, Berlin 1933, Bd 2, Tafel 34. Courtesy of Thüringer Universitäts-und Landesbibliothek, Friedrich Schiller University of Jena, Germany)

Friedrich Merkel (1845–1919). In 1875 he became assistant surgeon to Franz König (1832–1910) in Göttingen, Germany and subsequently studied surgery with Bernhard von Langenbeck (1810–1887). Riedel became Chief of the surgical department at the Städtisches Krankenhaus in Aachen, Northern Germany in 1882. Six years later he took up the Chair of Surgery and became Director of the surgical clinic at the University of Jena. Under his leadership the number of surgical referrals to the department steadily increased. When he retired in 1910 on account of ill health his department was performing more than 2000 operations annually.

Riedel was an energetic surgeon and a committed scientist. Before his appointment at Jena he had already published 36 articles and edited two editions of Franz König's *Textbook of General Surgery*. His interests were diverse and included such topics as development of the kidneys, lymphoedema after inguinal node dissection, and tuberculosis of the joints. Riedel was a pioneer in the surgical treatment of appendicitis

171

and cholecystitis, and is credited with performing the first choledochoduodenostomy in 1888. He is not only associated with Riedel's lobe but also with Riedel's thyroiditis, an uncommon chronic thyroiditis in which the gland is replaced by extensive fibrosis, which he described in 1896.

References

Gillard JH, Patel MC, Abrahams PH, Dixon AK. Riedel's lobe of the liver: fact or fiction? *Clin Anat* 1998;**11**:47–9.

James PM, Howard JM, Wolferth CC. Riedel's lobe of the liver. *Am J Surg* 1963;**105**:812–15.

Riedel B. Ueber den zungenförmigen Fortsatz des rechten Leberlappens und seine pathognostische Bedeutung für die Erkrankung der Gallenblase nebst Bemerkungen über Gallensteinoperationen. *Berliner Klinische Wochenschrift* 1888;**29**:577–81.

Sham R, Sain A, Silver L. Hypertrophic Riedel's lobe of the liver. *Clin Nucl Med* 1978;**3**:79–81.

Further reading

Obituary Bernhard Riedel. *Jenaische Zeitung* 16 September 1916.

Reitemeier RJ, Butt HR, Baggenstoss AH. Riedel's lobe of the liver. *Gastroenterology* 1958;**34**:1090–5.

Scheele S, Miller DA, Hardy KJ. The early operation for acute severe cholecystitis: the Riedel paper; an introduction and translation. *ANZ J Surg* 1999;**69**:871–3.

R Rokitansky–Aschoff sinus

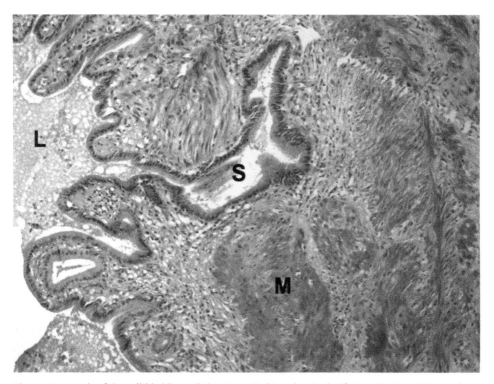

Photomicrograph of the gall bladder wall showing a Rokitansky–Aschoff sinus. S, sinus; M, muscle; L, lumen of gall bladder. Haematoxylin & eosin ×100. (Courtesy of Dr Jens Stahlschmidt, St James's University Hospital, Leeds, UK)

Rokitansky–Aschoff sinuses are epithelial outpouchings of gall bladder mucosa into and through the muscle layer of the gall bladder. They may sometimes be visible to the naked eye but are typically seen on microscopy. They can be found in normal adult gall bladders but are typically seen in association with cholelithiasis and cholecystitis. An exaggerated form of these sinuses occurs in adenomyomatosis of the gall bladder, when the outpouchings extend through the muscle layer of the gall bladder. The sinuses may then be visible by cholecystography or other imaging studies.

Rokitansky noted these outpouchings of gall bladder mucosa, which sometimes contained calculi, in his pathology text published in 1842. In a later publication in 1861 (von Rokitansky 1861), he elaborated further stating that the outpouchings of the mucosa were "...at times, in large number, usually of small size (millet and hempseed)." In 1905, Karl Aschoff presented a paper on cholelithiasis and cholecystitis based on his observations of 145 gall bladders, commenting that many gall bladders had epithelial invaginations that in some cases penetrated the muscle layer (Aschoff 1905). He believed that increased pressure within the lumen of the gall bladder from gallstones led to the formation and enlargement of these crypts.

For more than a century there has been confusion concerning the histological appearance, mode of formation, and pathological significance of these outpouchings, referred to as Rokitansky–Aschoff sinuses since 1927. Increased pressure within the gall bladder is almost certainly one aetiological factor. Rarely, the sinuses give rise to gall bladder cancer.

Carl von Rokitansky (1804–1878)

Rokitansky was born in Hradec Kràlové, now in the Czech Republic but then part of the Austrian empire. He became Professor of Pathology at Vienna General Hospital, where he personally performed more than 30,000 autopsies during his career. His contributions to pathology were numerous and far reaching. He was the first to demonstrate bacteria in the vegetations of endocarditis, to distinguish lobar from bronchopneumonia, and to describe spondylolisthesis. He made major advances in the understanding of congenital heart disease. One of his best known works, *Handbuch der pathologischen Anatomie*, was published in three volumes between 1842 and 1846.

Rokitansky received many honours. Most notably, he was President of the Academy of Sciences and was made a baron on his 70th birthday. As a consequence, he is sometimes referred to as Carl Freiherr von Rokitansky. Freiherr is a title meaning baron and not a middle name. Rokitansky was married with four sons, two of whom pursued musical careers like their mother and two became doctors.

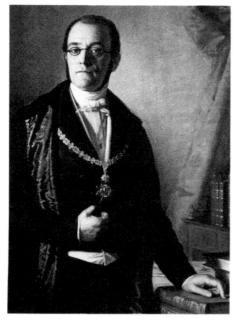

Carl von Rokitansky. (Courtesy of the Clendening History of Medicine Museum)

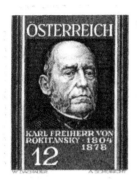

An Austrian postage stamp from a 1937 sequence featuring famous Austrian doctors. Rokitansky was again commemorated on an Austrian stamp in 1954, the 150th anniversary of his birth

Karl Albert Ludwig Aschoff (1866–1942)

Aschoff was an eminent German physician and pathologist who was Professor of Pathology at the University of Marburg from 1903 and at the University of Freiburg from 1906. It was at Freiburg that he established the internationally famous Institute of Pathology.

Aschoff's main interest was in cardiac pathology and physiology. Together with the Japanese pathologist, Sunao Tawara (1873–1952), he described the atrioventricular node in 1906. Aschoff also described the reticulendothelial system of phagocytic cells in the 1920s.

References

Aschoff L. Bemerkungen zur pathologischen Anatomie der Cholelithiasis und Cholecystitis. *Verh Deut Path Ges* 1905;**9**:41–8.

von Rokitansky C. *Handbuch der speciellen pathologischen Anatomie*. Braumüller und Seidel, Vienna 1842, Volume 2, p.374.

von Rokitansky CF. *Lehrbuch der pathologischen Anatomie*. W. Braumüller, Vienna, 1861, p.282.

Further reading

Albores-Saavedra J, Shukla D, Carrick K, Henson DE. In situ and invasive adenocarcinomas of the gallbladder extending into or arising from Rokitansky–Aschoff sinuses: a clinicopathologic study of 49 cases. *Am J Surg Pathol* 2004;**28**:621–8.

Gilder SSB. Carl von Rokitansky (1804–1878). *Canad M A J* 1954;**71**:70–2.

Klemperer P. Notes on Carl von Rokitansky's autobiography and inaugural address. *Bull Hist Med* 1961;**35**:374–80.

Lack EE, Albores-Saavedra J. *Pathology of the Pancreas, Gallbladder, Extrahepatic Biliary Tract, and Ampullary Region*. Oxford University Press US, New York, 2003, pp424–6.

Robertson HE, Ferguson WJ. The diverticula (Luschka's crypts) of the gallbladder. *Arch Pathol* 1945;**40**:312–33.

Rouvière's sulcus

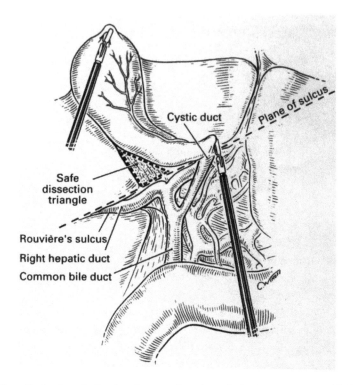

Diagram of Rouvière's sulcus, indicating the triangle within which dissection may safely be commenced in a plane ventral to that of the common bile duct. (From Hugh TB, Kelly MD, Mekisic A. Rouvière's sulcus: a useful landmark in laparoscopic cholecystectomy. *Br J Surg* 1997;**84**:1253–4. Fig.2, p.1253. © British Journal of Surgery Society Ltd. Reproduced with permission of John Wiley & Sons Ltd on behalf of the BJSS Ltd)

Various operative techniques have been described to minimise the risk of bile duct injury during laparoscopic cholecystectomy. Rouvière's sulcus is an anatomical landmark that some surgeons have found useful in identifying the plane of the common bile duct. This groove on the inferior surface of the right lobe of the liver runs for 2–5 cm to the right of the liver hilum. It usually contains the right portal triad or its branches. Henri Rouvière first described the sulcus in 1924 and noted that it was present in 81% of fetuses and infants and 52% of adults (Rouvière 1924). Subsequently, Couinaud found the sulcus in 73% of livers and highlighted its value in providing access to right portal structures during right-sided liver resections. Hugh et al (1997) identified the sulcus in 78% of patients at laparoscopic cholecystectomy and commented that gall bladder dissection could proceed safely in the triangle *ventral* to the plane of the sulcus when the gall bladder had been reflected cranially.

Numerous techniques have been reported to optimise safety in laparoscopic cholecystectomy, including lateral retraction of the gall bladder to open out the hepatobiliary triangle. However, if the surgeon decides to retract the gall bladder cranially, Rouvière's sulcus may be used to facilitate anatomical orientation before starting dissection of the gall bladder, which can then safely proceed up the gall bladder fossa.

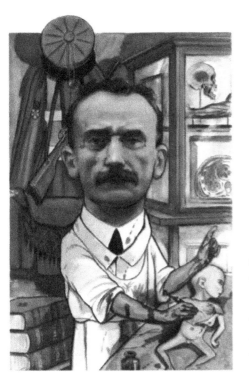

Caricature of Professor Henri Rouvière, Faculty of Medicine, Paris 1929 (*Chanteclair* No.254, 1/3/29)

*Chanteclair was a Parisian artistic and medical revue magazine issued between 1905 and 1935. Its circulation was mostly confined to the medical profession.

Henri Rouvière (1875–1952)

Rouvière was born at Le Bleymard in Southern France. He gained his medical doctorate from Montpellier in 1903. He joined the medical faculty of the University of Paris in 1910, becoming Professor of Anatomy in 1927. Many of his anatomical works are preserved in the Musée d'Anatomie Delmas-Orfila-Rouvière in Paris. He is also remembered by the Collège Henri Rouvière in his hometown of Le Bleymard.

Although Rouvière wrote several famous anatomy texts, he is best remembered for his detailed account of the anatomy of the human lymphatic system, which built upon the seminal work of the French anatomist Marie Sappey (1810–1896). Rouvière's node is the eponymous term sometimes used to refer to one of the lateral group of retropharyngeal lymph nodes at the base of the skull.

Rouvière's sulcus

References

Hugh TB, Kelly MD, Mekisic A. Rouvière's sulcus: a useful landmark in laparoscopic cholecystectomy. *Br J Surg* 1997;**84**:1253–4.

Rouvière H. Sur la configuration et la signification du sillon du processus caudé. *Bulletins et Memoires de la Societé Anatomique de Paris* 1924;**94**:355–8.

Further reading

Menegaux G. Henri Rouvière, 1875–1952. *Mémoires de l'Académie de Chirurgie* 1954;**80**:117–29.

Rouvière H. *Anatomie des Lymphatiques de l'Homme*. Masson, Paris, 1932.

Roux-en-Y jejunal anastomosis

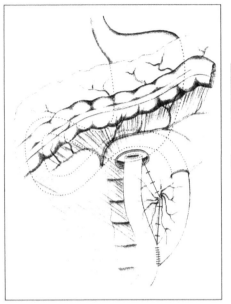
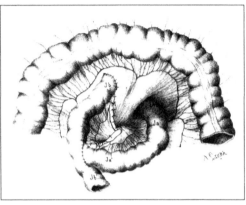

César Roux's original sketches of his Y jejunal anastomosis. (From Roux C. De la gastro-entérostomie. *Rev Gynécol Chir Abdom* 1897;1:67–122: plate 3, left ; and plate 2, right)

The Roux-en-Y jejunal anastomosis was originally devised for the treatment of antropyloric obstruction, which had hitherto been treated by partial gastrectomy and gastrojejunostomy, or pyloroplasty. César Roux first performed the procedure in January 1892 in a patient with an obstructing antropyloric tumour and later used the technique for bypassing malignant oesophagogastric obstruction. Roux acknowledged that he had not invented the Y anastomosis, which had been described in canine experiments by Wölfler, but carried out the procedure for the first time in a patient. The jejunum was transected 15–30 cm from the ligament of Treitz and a 10–12 cm limb of distal jejunum was brought up in a retrocolic position and anastomosed to the posterior wall of the stomach.

Postoperative hydration was achieved with subcutaneous or intravenous saline solutions and hypercaloric enemas. Oral feeding was commenced as early as the first day after surgery, the patient first being offered fluids in the form of water, milk, tea or even champagne! By 1900 Roux had performed 116 of these procedures but he abandoned its use for benign antropyloric obstruction in 1911, when he recognised that the problem of gastrojejunal anastomotic ulceration could be mitigated or prevented by the presence of bile and pancreatic juice with an end-to-side loop gastroenterostomy.

The Roux-en-Y jejunal anastomosis subsequently became popular as a versatile and effective reconstructive technique in upper gastrointestinal, hepatobiliary and pancreatic surgery.

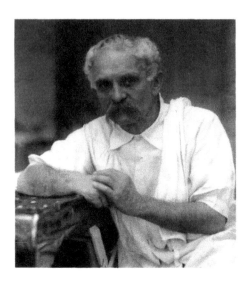

César Roux. (Anonymous. Collection of the Musée historique de Lausanne.)

César Roux (1857–1934)

Roux was the fifth son of French Huguenot immigrants to Switzerland. He initially intended to be a vet but was apparently put off by the students' uniform! He decided to study medicine and was supported financially by one of his brothers. At medical school in Bern he was greatly influenced by the eminent surgeon Theodor Kocher and by the pathologist Theodor Langhans. His doctoral thesis was on the anatomy of the anal musculature.

After graduation, on Kocher's advice Roux visited Vienna, Prague and Holland for further training before returning to Bern to become Kocher's first assistant. He then took up independent medical practice in Lausanne, where he was frequently assisted by his wife. Roux was appointed Professor of Surgery and Gynaecology at the newly founded University of Lausanne at the age of 33 years. Despite being described by Harvey Cushing, one of his many visitors, as "a rough diamond", Roux was hugely influential in the development of Swiss surgery.

Among his many contributions to surgery, he was one of the first to drain an appendiceal abscess (in 1883), he described the technique of jejunal interposition to repair the oesophagus in a child with a caustic oesophageal stricture, he described procedures to treat rectal prolapse and haemorrhoids, and, in February 1926, he performed the first adrenalectomy for a phaeochromocytoma.

Roux received numerous awards including the French Légion d'Honneur and honorary doctorates from the University of Chicago and the Sorbonne. He was made honorary mayor of Lausanne and Mont-la-Ville, and today there is a street named after him in Lausanne. However, he declined to accept honorary membership of the Royal College of Surgeons of England because he would have had to abandon his lectures in Lausanne for a few days! In later years he developed angina and died suddenly whilst consulting a patient.

References

Roux C. De la gastro-entérostomie. *Rev Gynécol Chir Abdom* 1897;**1**:67–122.

Further reading

Marion M. Notice nécrologique sur M. Cesar Roux (de Lausanne) (1857–1934). *Bull Acad Med Paris* 1935;**113**:123–6.

Roux C. Chirurgie gastrointestinale. *Rev Chir* 1893;**13**:402–3.

Roux C. Les anastomoses intestinales et gastrointestinales. *Rev Gynécol Chir Abdom* 1900;**4**:787–96.

Vauthey JN, Maddern GJ, Gertsch P. Cesar Roux – Swiss pioneer in surgery. *Surgery* 1992;**112**:946–50.

Wood M. Eponyms in biliary tract surgery. *Am J Surg* 1979;**138**:746–54.

S | Saint's triad

Saint's triad is the concurrence of gallstones, hiatal hernia, and diverticular disease in a patient.

Saint never published the triad, which was attributed to him in a paper written in 1948 by one of his ex-students, C.J.B. Muller, a radiologist at Johannesburg General Hospital: "During last year Professor Saint of Cape Town mentioned to me during a discussion about double pathology, the association of hiatus hernia, sacculi of the colon and gall-stones. Its prognostic importance in avoiding unwarranted treatment, and the wide differential diagnosis from a host of pulmonary, cardiac and abdominal conditions, makes the triad of practical as well as of academic interest." (Muller 1948)

One early report of 170 adult patients with hiatus hernia followed up over several years found that 14% had evidence of Saint's triad (Palmer 1955). There is no commonly accepted pathophysiological basis for the coexistence of the triad although Denis Burkitt (1911–1993) suggested that a lack of dietary fibre resulted in all three conditions. Some authors have disputed the association and others have suggested that it is simply a result of each being a common Western disease.

Perhaps the real merit of Saint's triad lies in the importance he placed on considering the possibility of multiple separate diseases to explain a patient's clinical signs and symptoms. This is the antithesis of Occam's razor, which states that "plurality must not be posited without necessity" (after William of Ockham, a fourteenth century English logician and Franciscan friar).

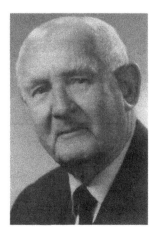

Charles Saint. (Courtesy of Groote Schuur Hospital, Cape Town, South Africa)

Charles F.M. Saint (1886–1973)

Born in Northumberland, England, he graduated from the University of Durham in 1908 and served as Rutherford Morison's assistant. After meritorious service as a surgeon in World War I, for which he was awarded the Commander of the British Empire and the Médaille d'Honneur, he took up a position as the first Professor

183

of Surgery at the University of Cape Town, South Africa. He remained there from 1920 until 1946. He was greatly revered by his students and fellow surgeons and was famous for his aphorisms such as "Early to bed and early to rise: work like hell but organize".

Saint retired to the island of Sark in the Channel Isles at the age of 60 years, adamant that a surgeon should retire before his skill diminishes.

References

Muller CJB. Hiatus hernia, diverticula and gall stones; Saint's triad. *S Afr Med J* 1948;**22**:376–82.

Palmer ED. Saint's triad (hiatus hernia, gall stones and diverticulosis coli): the problem of properly directing surgical therapy. *Am J Dig Dis* 1955;**22**:314–15.

Further reading

Anon. In memoriam. Charles F M Saint, CBE, FRCS (1886–1973). *Br J Surg* 1973;**60**:407.

Burkitt DP, Walker AR. Saint's triad: confirmation and explanation. *S Afr Med J* 1976;**50**:2136–8.

Saint CF. Saint's triad. The origin and story of its recognition. *Rev Surg* 1966;**23**:1–4

Schulenburg CAR. In memoriam Charlie F M Saint CBE MD MS FRCSEng FRACS. *S Afr Med J* 1973;**47**:286b.

Duct of Santorini

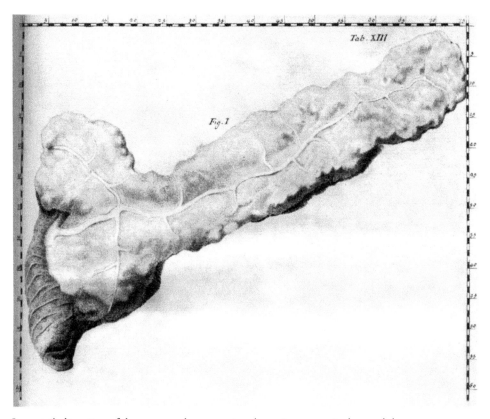

Santorini's dissection of the pancreas demonstrating the main pancreatic duct and the accessory pancreatic duct opening into the duodenum above. (From Girardi M. Jo: *Dominico Santorini Anatomici Summi Septemdecim Tabulae*. Ex Regia Typographia, Parmae, Tabula XIII, p. 1775. By kind permission of the Mayo Foundation for Medical Education & Research)

Santorini's *Observationes Anatomicae* was published in 1724 (Santorini 1724). He planned to include his discovery of the accessory pancreatic duct in a second edition of this text but he died before completing the project. Fortunately, his material was collected and published in 1775 by his disciple Michael Girardi, Professor of Anatomy in Parma, Italy. *Anatomici Summi-Septemdecim Tabulae* ('the excellent anatomist's seventeen drawings') contains a clear illustration of the pancreas and its accessory duct (Santorini 1775). Santorini named the latter the 'upper pancreatic duct'. He noted that the lower main pancreatic duct opened into the duodenum at the 'greater caruncle'. According to Girardi, Santorini performed several hundred pancreatic dissections with the aid of a magnifying glass. His illustrations were produced with the help of the artist Giovanni Battista Piazzetta and the engraver Florentia Marcella. Remarkably, they were drawn to scale.

185

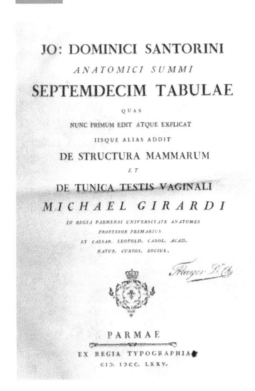

JO: DOMINICI SANTORINI

ANATOMICI SUMMI

SEPTEMDECIM TABULAE

QUAS

NUNC PRIMUM EDIT ATQUE EXPLICAT

IISQUE ALIAS ADDIT

DE STRUCTURA MAMMARUM

ET

DE TUNICA TESTIS VAGINALI

MICHAEL GIRARDI

IN REGIA PARMENSI UNIVERSITATE ANATOMES
PROFESSOR PRIMARIUS
ET CAESAR. LEOPOLD. CAROL. ACAD.
NATUR. CURIOS. SOCIUS.

PARMAE

EX REGIA TYPOGRAPHIA
CIƆ. IƆCC. LXXV.

Title page of Santorini's *Anatomici Summi-Septemdecim Tabulae* published posthumously in 1775, 38 years after his death.* (By permission of the Mayo Foundation for Medical Education and Research)

*A first edition of this text sold for nearly $6000 at Christies in New York in 2007.

An embryological explanation of the accessory pancreatic duct (and of pancreas divisum) was not provided until 1812, when Johann Frederich Meckel (1781–1833) reported that the pancreas is derived from fusion of dorsal and ventral primordia in the embryo. According to Stern (1986), Johannes Rhode (1587–1656) was probably the first to identify an accessory pancreatic duct in 1646 in Padua in a female cadaver but his description was not published until 1661. Double human pancreatic ducts were subsequently described by others including Regnier de Graaf (1664), Frederik Ruysch (1665), and Samuel Collins (1685) but these were generally considered anomalous. There were numerous descriptions of the gross anatomy of the pancreas in the seventeenth century and Santorini was probably aware of some of these but he was the first to recognise the accessory duct as a normal variant. According to Suarez (1981), Santorini also described papillary valves, mucosal folds within the major duodenal papilla.

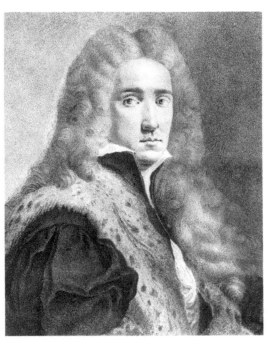

Giovanni Domenico Santorini (1681–1727). (From Girardi M. Jo: *Dominico Santorini Anatomici Summi Septemdecim Tabulae*. Ex Regia Typographia, Parmae, p.1775. By kind permission of the Mayo Foundation for Medical Education & Research)

Giovanni Domenico Santorini (1681–1737)

Born in Venice, the son of an apothecary, Santorini rejected the Jesuit priesthood and law as possible careers and chose to become a physician, obtaining his medical degree from Pisa University in 1701. He was a pupil of the famous Marcello Malpighi (1628–1694), the Italian histologist, anatomist, physiologist and physician who, among his many discoveries, identified the existence of capillaries.

Santorini was appointed Incisore di Anatomia (anatomy prosector) in Venice at just 23 years of age. The office of anatomist was divided between that of Incisore, who prepared specimens, and Lettore, whose responsibility it was to demonstrate the anatomy to medical doctors. At this time, corpses of criminals were dissected by permission of the Prince. Santorini was renowned for his detailed dissections and he rapidly assumed the roles of both Incisore and Lettore (Cagnetto 1916).

His other anatomical studies included the muscles of facial expression, the corniculate cartilages of the larynx, and the nasal conchae. He became *protomedicus* (chief physician) at the Spedaletto Hospital in Venice where he also taught obstetrics. Santorini's scientific approach to anatomy and medicine is illustrated by his publication on fevers in which he was sceptical of contemporary remedies such as an extract of Spring vipers as advocated by a fellow anatomist, Giovanni Battista Morgagni (1682–1771), recommending plenty of fluids instead (Santorini 1734). He died from an infective illness, which may have been contracted from a cadaver.

References

Cagnetto G. *Un Grande Anatomico della Serenissima (Giandomenico Santorini)*. Atti del Reale Instituto Veneto di Scienze 1915–16. Carlo Ferrari, Venezia, Tomo LXXV:1163–1188.

Rhodius J. *Mantissa anatomica, extat cum Thomam Bartholinum historiarum anatomicar and medicar rarior.* Centuria V and VI. Typis Henrici Godiani, Hafniae, 1661 (Cambridge University Library).

Santorini G. *Istruzione introno alle Febbri.* Giovambattista Recurti, Venezia, 1734.

Santorini GD. *Observationes Anatomicae.* Giovanni Battista Recurti, Venetiis, 1724.

Santorini GD. *Anatomici Summi Septemdecim Tabulae.* Ex Regia Typographia, Parmae, 1775.

Stern CD. A historical perspective on the discovery of the accessory duct of the pancreas, the ampulla 'of Vater' and *pancreas divisum. Gut* 1986;**27**:203–12.

Further reading

Flati G, Andren-Sandberg A. Wirsung and Santorini: the men behind the ducts. *Pancreatology* 2002;**2**:4–11.

Wood M. Eponyms in biliary tract surgery. *Am J Surg* 1979;**138**:746–54.

TRAITÉ

D'ANATOMIE

DESCRIPTIVE

AVEC FIGURES INTERCALÉES DANS LE TEXTE

PAR

PH. C. SAPPEY

Professeur d'anatomie a la Faculté de médecine de Paris
Membre de l'Académie de médecine

Deuxième édition entièrement refondue

TOME QUATRIÈME

SPLANCHNOLOGIE

PARIS

ADRIEN DELAHAYE, LIBRAIRE-ÉDITEUR
PLACE DE L'ÉCOLE-DE-MÉDECINE
1874

Tous droits réservés.

Title page from Sappey's 1874 book. (From Sappey MPC. *Traité d'Anatomie Descriptive*. Volume 4: *Splanchnologie*. Adrien Delahaye, Paris, 1874

Sappey's veins are veins within the falciform ligament that become dilated in portal hypertension. Sappey observed these veins in postmortem livers from subjects with advanced cirrhosis and portal hypertension. He considered them to be relatively insignificant in normal individuals but noted that they become markedly dilated in portal hypertension, when they act as portosystemic conduits. In Volume 4 of his *Traité d'Anatomie Descriptive* published in 1874, he described five groups of 'accessory portal veins' (Sappey 1874). However, in a later publication in 1883 (Sappey 1883), he had refined the classification into superior and inferior veins within the falciform ligament. The superior ones extended from the median part of the diaphragm to the convex surface of the liver, where they anastomosed with peripheral branches of the portal vein within the liver. The inferior group ran between periumbilical and epigastric veins and the umbilical recess. Occasionally, they anastomosed with the left portal vein or a patent segment of the umbilical vein. He also noted that when very dilated, these veins could be associated with a palpable thrill and an audible venous hum.

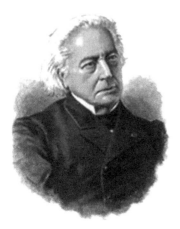

Marie Philibert Constant Sappey.

Marie Philibert Constant Sappey (1810–1896)

Sappey was a leading French nineteenth century anatomist. He graduated in medicine from the University of Paris in 1843, and went on to hold the Chair of Anatomy between 1868 and 1886. He was elected President of the French Academy of Medicine in 1887.

His *Traité d'Anatomie Descriptive* was published in four volumes between 1847 and 1874 and *Anatomie, Physiologie, Pathologie des Vaisseaux Lymphatiques Considerées Chez l'homme et Les Vertébres* in 1874 (Sappey 1874). Using mercury injections in cadavers, he produced wonderfully detailed illustrations of the lymph drainage of the skin. The term 'Sappey's plexus' has been used to describe the network of lymphatics in the areola of the nipple.

References

Sappey MPC. *Traité d'Anatomie Descriptive*. Volume 4: *Splanchnologie*. Adrien Delahaye, Paris, 1874, pp329–31.

Sappey MC. Mémoire sur les veines portes accessoires. *Journal de l'Anatomie et de la Physiologie Normales et Pathologiques de l'Homme et des Animaux.* 1883;**19**:517–25.

Further reading

Arvy L, Rivet R. Marie Philibert Constant Sappey (1810–1896). The man and the lymphologist. *Bull Assoc Anat* 1976;**60**:63–79.

Martin BF, Tudor RG. The umbilical and paraumbilical veins of man. *J Anat* 1980;**130**:305–22.

Sengstaken–Blakemore tube

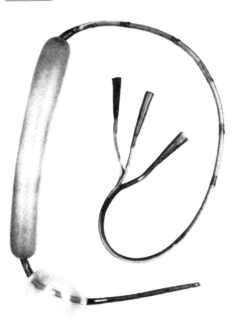

BALLOON TAMPONAGE FOR THE CONTROL OF HEMORRHAGE
FROM ESOPHAGEAL VARICES*

ROBERT W. SENGSTAKEN, M.D., AND ARTHUR H. BLAKEMORE, M.D.

NEW YORK, N. Y.

FROM THE PRESBYTERIAN HOSPITAL OF NEW YORK CITY

The Sengstaken–Blakemore tube (top) as shown in the original 1950 publication (bottom). (From Sengstaken RW, Blakemore AH. Balloon tamponage for the control of hemorrhage from esophageal varices. *Ann Surg* 1950;**131**:781–9, Fig.1, p.784 © Lippincott, Williams & Wilkins)

This triple lumen rubber tube developed by two New York surgeons, Sengstaken and Blakemore, in 1946 was designed to arrest bleeding from ruptured oesophageal varices, typically in patients with cirrhosis of the liver. Around the larger central nasogastric lumina used for drainage and feeding, there were two smaller lumena connected to gastric and oesophageal balloons. Once the gastric balloon was inflated with 150–200 ml of air, traction on the tube compressed the gastro-oesophageal junction and its submucosal varices. The oesophageal balloon was inflated with air to a pressure of around 20–25 mm of mercury. A key feature was reinforcement of the rubber of the oesophageal balloon to prevent it from becoming deformed and migrating into the stomach, a modification that Blakemore modestly credited to Sengstaken in a later publication. Deep sedation or general anaesthesia was usually necessary to subdue the patient's retching reflexes. The tube was deflated after 48 hours to see if bleeding had stopped, and reinflated if necessary. In patients needing prolonged tamponade (which the authors called 'tamponage'), enteral feeding could be given via the nasogastric lumen.

Sengstaken and Blakemore acknowledged that they were not the first to use this technique, but the specific design of the tube was new. In their paper, they reported the successful use of the tube in 30 patients with bleeding oesophageal varices.

191

S

Modifications to both the tube and its use were subsequently reported. For example, the Linton–Nachlas tube had only a gastric balloon but included a lumen to drain the oesophagus; this aimed to avoid the complication of oesophageal ulceration from the oesophageal balloon (Linton 1953; Nachlas 1955). Later, the King's College Hospital group highlighted some of the pitfalls of balloon tamponade such as accidentally inflating the gastric balloon in the oesophagus, causing oesophageal rupture or the consequences of excessive mechanical traction (Vlavianos et al 1989). With the availability of modern endoscopic techniques* and interventional radiology, the Sengstaken–Blakemore tube and its derivatives are less often used today but still have a place in the emergency management of intractable bleeding from oesophageal varices.

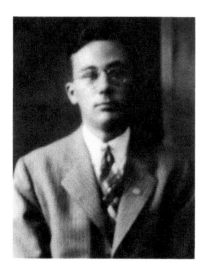

Robert Sengstaken. Photograph taken in 1943. (Courtesy of Archives and Special Collections, Columbia University Health Sciences Library)

*Endoscopic injection sclerotherapy of oesophageal varices via a rigid oesophagoscope was first reported by two Swedish surgeons, Crafoord and Frenckner in 1939 but the application of the technique was overshadowed by the development of portosystemic shunt surgery. Not until the 1970s, with the advent of fibreoptic endoscopy and the development of better sclerosants, was endoscopic injection sclerotherapy used routinely. In 1988, Van Stiegmann and Goff introduced endoscopic variceal ligation as an alternative to sclerotherapy.

Robert W. Sengstaken (1923–1978)

Sengstaken graduated from Columbia University College of Physicians and Surgeons in 1946, after serving in the Navy during World War II. He trained in surgery at the Presbyterian Hospital, New York, initially with Arthur Blakemore, but subsequently at Columbia University's Neurological Institute. He became Chief of Neurosurgery at

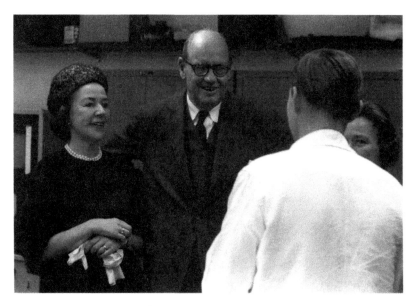

Arthur Blakemore (centre). Photograph by Elizabeth Wilcox taken in 1963 at the opening of the Arthur H. Blakemore Laboratory for Vascular Research, Columbia University College of Physicians and Surgeons, New York. (Courtesy of Archives and Special Collections, Columbia University Health Sciences Library)

St Charles Hospital in Long Island and was Associate Professor of Clinical Surgery at the State University of New York at Stony Brook, Long Island. Of the three literature citations on PubMed listed for 'Sengstaken RW', one relates to the Sengstaken–Blakemore tube, one to general surgery, and one to neurosurgery. He died of a heart attack at just 54 years of age, survived by his wife and five children.

Arthur Hendley Blakemore (1897–1970)

Blakemore was born in Virginia and obtained his MD from Johns Hopkins University, Baltimore in 1922. He was on the staff at Columbia University College of Physicians and Surgeons in New York from 1929 until he retired in 1962, and also worked at the Presbyterian Hospital. During World War II, Blakemore served as Director of the National Research Council, researching vascular repair after trauma. He became an international authority on the surgery of portal hypertension but is also known for his work on abdominal aortic aneurysm. He was a fellow of many surgical societies and President of the Society for Vascular Surgery. On his retirement from Columbia University College of Physicians and Surgeons, a laboratory for the study of hepatic circulation was named in his honour.

193

References

Crafoord C, Frenckner P. New surgical treatment of varicose veins of the oesophagus. *Acta Otolaryngo* 1939;**27**:422–9.

Linton RR. The emergency and definitive treatment of bleeding esophageal varices. *Gastroenterology* 1953;**24**:1–9.

Nachlas MM. A new triple-lumen tube for the diagnosis and treatment of upper gastrointestinal hemorrhage. *N Engl J Med* 1955;**252**:720–1.

Sengstaken RW, Blakemore AH. Balloon tamponage for the control of hemorrhage from esophageal varices. *Ann Surg* 1950;**131**:781–9.

Van Stiegmann G, Goff JS. Endoscopic esophageal varix ligation: preliminary clinical experience. *Gastrointest Endosc* 1988;**34**:113–17.

Vlavianos P, Gimson AE, Westaby D, Williams R. Balloon tamponade in variceal bleeding: use and misuse. *BMJ* 1989;**298**:1158.

Further reading

Anon. Arthur Blakemore, Surgeon and Teacher, Dead. *New York Times* Oct 10, 1970.

Anon. Dr Robert W Sengstaken, 54, a Neurosurgeon on L.I. *New York Times* Jan 9, 1978.

Blakemore AH. Treatment of bleeding esophageal varices with balloon tamponage. *N Y State J Med* 1954;**54**:2057–85.

Spiegel lobe

The Spiegel lobe is usually synonymous with the caudate lobe of the liver. Although named after Spiegel, he was probably not the first to describe this anatomic entity. Some authors, including Couinaud, consider Spiegel's lobe to represent only part of the caudate lobe (segment I), the other part being the paracaval portion (segment IX). Spiegel also described the semilunar line alongside the rectus abdominis muscle after which Spiegelian hernias are named.

His writings include two posthumous publications, *De Formato Foetu* (1626) and *De Humani Corporis Fabrica Libri Decem* (1627).

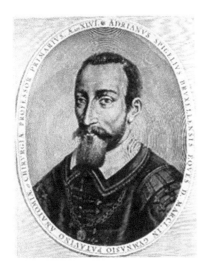

Adriaan van der Spiegel.

Adriaan van der Spiegel (1578–1625)

Also known as Adrian van der Spieghel and, in Latin, Adrianus Spigelius. Spiegel was an anatomist, physician and botanist. Born in Brussels, Belgium, he was descended from a line of Flemish surgeons. He attended the universities of Louvain, Leiden, and Padua, graduating in medicine in 1603. In 1612 he left Italy and travelled through Belgium and Germany before settling in Moravia. In 1616 he was appointed Professor of Anatomy and Surgery in Padua, where he was renowned for his public performances in the famous anatomy theatre.

References

van der Spiegel A, Casseri G. *De Formato Foetu*. GB Martini & L Pasquatus, Padua,1626.

van der Spiegel A, Casseri D, Bucretius D *et al. De Humani Corporis Fabrica Libri Decem*. Evangelista Deuchino, Venice, 1627.

Spiegel lobe

Further reading

Couinaud C. Dorsal sector of the liver. *Chirurgie* 1998;**123**:8–15.

Jassem W, Heaton ND, Rela M. Reducing bile leak following segmental liver transplantation: understanding biliary anatomy of the caudate lobe. *Am J Transpl* 2008;**8**:271–4.

Skandalakis PN, Zoras O, Skandalakis JE, Mirilas P. Spigelian hernia: surgical anatomy, embryology, and technique of repair. *Am Surg* 2006;**72**:42–8.

S Sugiura devascularisation procedure

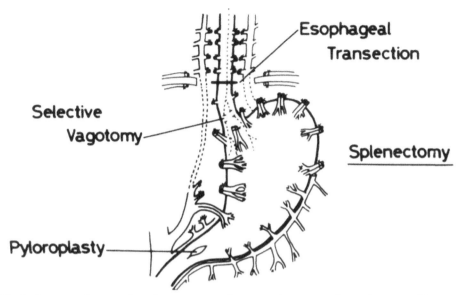

The Sugiura procedure: esophageal transection with paraesophagogastric devascularisation. (From Sugiura M, Futagawa S. A new technique for treating esophageal varices. *J Thorac Cardiovasc Surg* 1973;**66**:677–85, Fig. 1, p.678 © Elsevier)

The Sugiura procedure is a devascularisation technique for treating portal hypertension. The procedure consists of two operations that may be carried out in one or two stages. Firstly, via a left lateral thoracotomy, the distal oesophagus is thoroughly devascularised up to the level of the inferior pulmonary vein. The anterior half of the oesophagus is then transected at the level of the diaphragm and reanastomosed with some 70–90 interrupted sutures to occlude the varices in its wall. Secondly, via an upper midline incision with left lateral extension, a splenectomy is performed and the abdominal oesophagus, cardia, and proximal half of the stomach are devascularised. Because of the vagotomy, a pyloroplasty is added to complete the operation.

The aim of the Sugiura procedure was to prevent bleeding from oesophageal varices without impairing hepatic portal blood flow, which would expose the cirrhotic patient to the risk of hepatic encephalopathy. The operation was widely applied in Japan with low operative mortality and re-bleeding rates. However, the technique was not very popular in the West, perhaps because of higher perioperative morbidity and mortality rates or because of the availability and interest in alternative approaches. Devascularisation procedures tended to be reserved for patients with complications from portal hypertension who could not be managed by endoscopic therapy and who were not candidates for a portosystemic shunt, transjugular intrahepatic portosystemic shunt, or liver transplantation.

The Sugiura procedure has been used in children and adults. In 1984, Sugiura and Futagawa reported a personal series of 671 patients who had undergone the procedure, three-quarters of whom had cirrhosis (Sugiura and Fatagawa 1984). In elective cases, the operative mortality was less than 4% and the incidence of recurrent bleeding only 1.5%. Numerous modifications of the original procedure have been reported such as access via a single thoracoabdominal or abdominal incision, oesophageal transection using a circular stapler, avoidance of splenectomy, and an endoscopic approach but the general principles remain unchanged.

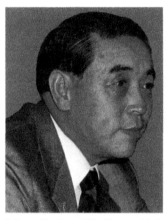

Mitsuo Sugiura. (Kindly provided by Professor A Yamataka, Juntendo University School of Medicine, Tokyo)

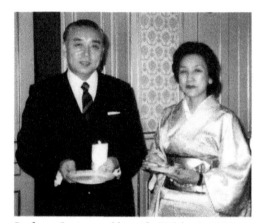

Professor Sugiura and his wife, Hideko, in 1985. (Kindly provided by Professor A Yamataka, Juntendo University School of Medicine, Tokyo)

Mitsuo Sugiura (1926–1988)

Sugiura was a Japanese surgeon at Juntendo University in Tokyo. He graduated from the University of Tokyo in 1950, obtained a PhD from the same institution in 1958, and was appointed Professor of Surgery at Juntendo University School of Medicine in 1979. Five years later he became Chairman of Surgery and Vice Director. His major research interest was the surgical management of portal hypertension, a subject on which he was a worldwide authority. On his retirement in 1990, he was succeeded by his colleague, collaborator, and co-author, Shunji Futagawa. Sugiura suffered a myocardial infarction whilst operating and died at the age of 62 years.

References

Sugiura M, Futagawa S. A new technique for treating esophageal varices. *J Thorac Cardiovasc Surg* 1973;**66**:677–85.

Sugiura M, Futagawa S. Esophageal transection with paraesophagogastric devascularizations (the Sugiura procedure) in the treatment of esophageal varices. *World J Surg* 1984;**8**:673–82.

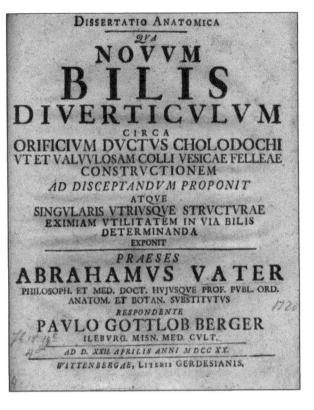

DISSERTATIO ANATOMICA
QVA
NOVVM
BILIS
DIVERTICVLVM
CIRCA
ORIFICIVM DVCTVS CHOLODOCHI
VT ET VALVVLOSAM COLLI VESICAE FELLEAE
CONSTRVCTIONEM
AD DISCEPTANDVM PROPONIT
ATQVE
SINGVLARIS VTRIVSQVE STRVCTVRAE
EXIMIAM VTILITATEM IN VIA BILIS
DETERMINANDA
EXPONIT
PRAESES
ABRAHAMVS VATER
PHILOSOPH. ET MED. DOCT. HVJVSQVE PROF. PVBL. ORD.
ANATOM. ET BOTAN. SVBSTITVTVS
RESPONDENTE
PAVLO GOTTLOB BERGER
ILEBVRG. MISN. MED. CVLT.
AD D. XXII. APRILIS ANNI MDCC XX.
WITTENBERGAE, LITERIS GERDESIANIS,

Title page of Vater's 1720 manuscript describing the hepatopancreatic ampulla (Vater 1720). (Courtesy of the Universitaetsbibliothek Tübingen)

In 1720, Abraham Vater described a tubercle or elevation of the mucosa in the duodenum where the biliary and pancreatic ducts came together. He recognised that there was no simple union of the two ducts: "those double ducts that come together in no single combination". Vater used an injection technique developed by the Dutch anatomist, Frederick Ruysch (1638–1731) to demonstrate that the bile and pancreatic juice mixed within the tubercle. The title page of his original report *Treatise on a new diverticulum near the orifice of the common bile duct and also on the valvular arrangement in the neck of the gallbladder, both very important structures for the passage of bile* had two authors, Abraham Vater and Paul Gottlob Berger. However, the Vater–Berger diverticulum subsequently became known only as the ampulla of Vater after Albrecht von Haller (1708–1777) referred to it in this way in his *Bibliotheca Anatomica* published in the 1770s.

According to Velasco-Suarez (1981), the ampulla of Vater had been described previously by Santorini. Stern (1986) states that Samuel Collins (1618–1710), anatomist and Fellow of the College of Physicians in London, had provided an even earlier description of the ampulla in 1685 but Collins really described the duodenal papilla rather than the ampulla (Collins 1685).

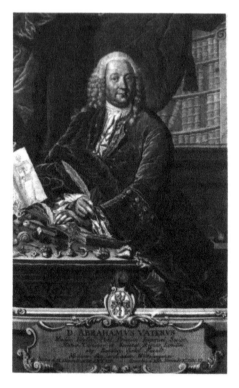

Abraham Vater. (Courtesy of Archiv der Deutschen
Akademie der Naturforscher Leopoldina, Halle).

Abraham Vater (1684–1751)

Abraham Vater, the son of a distinguished German doctor, was born in Wittenberg,
Germany, where he studied at the University, obtaining a degree in philosophy in
1706. After further studies in Leipzig he gained his medical degree in 1710. He then
travelled to Germany, England, and Holland and it was while visiting the famous
Dutch anatomist, Frederik Ruysch (1638–1731) in Amsterdam that he learnt to
prepare anatomical specimens from cadavers.

After returning to Wittenberg in 1719, he was appointed Professor of Anatomy
and Botany. He founded an anatomy museum, opened up anatomy demonstrations
to women as well as men, and managed to procure the corpses of suicide victims for
dissection. In 1737 he also became Professor of Pathology and, nine years later, was
appointed to the Chair of Therapeutics, which was considered the highest academic
position at the time. He was deeply interested in alchemy but in keeping with the
art, destroyed the records of his experiments.

In addition to the hepatopancreatic ampulla, Vater described a duct in the embryo
that connects the thyroid diverticulum to the posterior part of the tongue (Vater's
duct), and sensory end organs in the skin consisting of concentric layers of connective
tissue surrounding a nerve ending (Vater–Pacini corpuscles). He also wrote papers

200

on smallpox vaccination, popularising a technique in which a small amount of pus taken from a skin lesion of a patient with mild disease was used to inoculate a naive recipient (more than 70 years before Edward Jenner's experiments with cowpox). Vater was a member of the German Academy of Medicine for 43 years.

References

Collins S. *A Systeme of Anatomy, Treating of the Body of Man, Beasts, Birds, Fish, Insects, and Plants.* Thomas Newcombe, London, 1685.

Stern CD. A historical perspective on the discovery of the accessory duct of the pancreas, the ampulla 'of Vater' and *pancreas divisum. Gut* 1986;**27**:203–12.

Vater A, Berger PG. *Dissertatio Anatomica qua Novum Bilis Diverticulum circa Orificium Ductus Choledochi ut et Valvulosam Colli Vesicae Felleae Constructionem ad Disceptandum Proponit.* Literis Gerdesianis, Wittenbergae, 1720.

Velasco-Suarez C. The Santorini valves. *Mt Sinai J Med* 1981;**48**:149–57.

Further reading

Boyden EA. The pars intestinalis of the common bile duct, as viewed by the older anatomists (Vesalius, Glisson, Bianchi, Vater, Haller, Santorini etc.). *Anat Rec* 1936;**66**:217–32.

Wood M. Eponyms in biliary tract surgery. *Am J Surg* 1979;**138**:746–54.

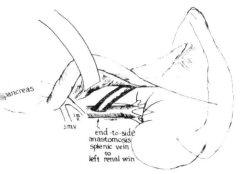

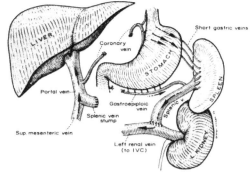

The distal splenorenal shunt as shown in Warren's original 1967 paper. (Reproduced with permission from Warren WD, Zeppa R, Fomon JJ. Selective trans-splenic decompression of gastroesophageal varices by distal splenorenal shunt. *Ann Surg* 1967;**166**:437–55, Fig.8, p.443. © Lippincott, Williams & Wilkins).

A more comprehensive illustration of the distal splenorenal shunt. (From Smith RB, Warren WD. Selective distal splenorenal shunt for bleeding esophageal varices. *Ann Rev Med* 1975;**26**:229–34. Reprinted with permission from *Annual Review of Medicine*, Volume 26 © 1975 by Annual Reviews www.annualreviews.org).

Dean Warren pioneered the development of the distal splenorenal shunt (later synonymous with the 'Warren shunt') for the treatment of portal hypertension. He first described the shunt with colleagues, Robert Zeppa and John Fomon in 1967, when he was Professor and Chairman of Surgery at the University of Miami (Warren et al 1967). At that time, portocaval shunts were commonly performed to treat variceal bleeding from portal hypertension but they were associated with a high incidence of hepatic failure. Warren's aim was to create a shunt that allowed continued portal perfusion of the hepatic parenchyma and yet decompressed gastro-oesophageal varices enough to prevent recurrent variceal bleeding. Proof of concept was first established in dogs with portal hypertension induced by an arteriovenous shunt.

In the original 1967 description, the distal splenorenal shunt was combined with partial gastric devascularisation. Portal vein thrombus was a potential complication but in most cases when this occurred, it resolved without progression to portal vein occlusion. The superiority of this shunt over portocaval shunts for patients with cirrhotic portal hypertension and bleeding oesophageal varices was confirmed in a prospective randomised, controlled clinical trial reported in 1978 (Rikkers et al 1978). Cumulative results in the 1970s and 1980s showed a perioperative mortality rate of less than 5% and a shunt patency rate of greater than 90%. With the advent of liver transplantation and transjugular intrahepatic portosystemic shunts, the use of surgical portosystemic shunts for portal hypertension secondary to cirrhosis declined

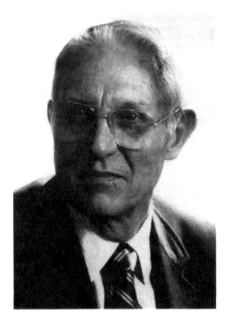

Dean Warren. (Reproduced with permission of the Department of Surgery, Emory University School of Medicine)

but the distal splenorenal shunt remains a useful option in selected patients with refractory portal hypertension.

W. Dean Warren (1924–1989)

Warren was born in Miami, Florida. After serving in the US Marine Corps during World War II he graduated from Johns Hopkins School of Medicine in 1950, where he began his surgical career. He completed his surgical training at the University of Michigan, Ann Arbor, and St Louis, Missouri. After finishing his residency in 1955, he began his studies on portal hypertension.

In 1963 he took up the Chair of Surgery at the University of Miami and, in 1971, he moved to Emory University School of Medicine in Atlanta, Georgia, where he was Joseph Brown Whitehead Professor of Surgery and Chairman of Surgery until his death in 1989.

In addition to his lifelong studies of portal hypertension, Warren was also interested in surgical training and education (the subject of his presidential address to the American Surgical Association in 1983) and in the application of randomised, controlled clinical trials in surgery. Among his many awards and achievements, Warren was president of the American Surgical Association (1983), the American College of Surgeons (1986), the Southern Surgical Association, and the Society of University Chairmen. He was married with one son and four daughters.

References

Rikkers LF, Rudman D, Galambos JT, et al. A randomized, controlled trial of distal splenorenal shunt. *Ann Surg* 1978;**188**:271–82.

Smith RB, Warren WD. Selective distal splenorenal shunt for bleeding esophageal varices. *Ann Rev Med* 1975;**26**:229–34.

Warren WD, Zeppa R, Fomon JJ. Selective trans-splenic decompression of gastroesophageal varices by distal splenorenal shunt. *Ann Surg* 1967;**166**:437–55.

Further reading

Portal hypertension. W. Dean Warren, MD, Memorial issue. *Am J Surg* 1990;**160**:1–138.

Warren WD. Controlled Clinical Research: Opportunities and Problems for the Surgeon. Presidential Address, Society for Surgery of the Alimentary Tract, 1973. *Am J Surg* 1974;**127**:3–8.

Warren WD. Not for the Profession...for the People. Presidential Address, American Surgical Association, 1983. *Ann Surg* 1983;**198**:241–50.

Warren WD, Millikan WJ, Henderson JM, et al. Ten years' portal hypertensive surgery at Emory. *Ann Surg* 1982;**195**:530–41.

Zeppa R. W. Dean Warren, MD October 28, 1924–May 10, 1989. *Arch Surg* 1989;**124**:767–8.

W Whipple pancreaticoduodenectomy/ Whipple's triad

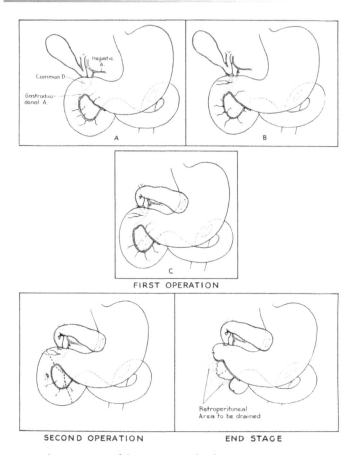

Consecutive steps in the two stages of the pancreaticoduodenectomy operation. (Reproduced from Whipple AO, Parsons WB, Mullins CR. Treatment of carcinoma of the ampulla of Vater. *Ann Surg* 1935;**102**:763–79. Fig.2, p.765. © Lippincott, Williams & Wilkins)

Early in 1934, Whipple performed a biliary bypass operation (choledochoduodenostomy and cholecystostomy), followed by local excision of a periampullary pancreatic cancer. In this procedure, he re-implanted the common bile duct and pancreatic remnant into the duodenal wall using catgut sutures. The patient died two days later from dehiscence of the pancreaticoduodenal anastomosis. A second patient with a periampullary carcinoma, operated on in August 1934, fared better; this time Whipple constructed a preliminary cholecystogastrostomy and then carried out a pancreaticoduodenectomy using fine silk sutures to perform the duodenal anastomosis. The patient developed stenosis of the cholecystogastrostomy and recurrent disease and eventually died from cholangitis nine months later.

Whipple's first truly successful pancreaticoduodenectomy was performed in 1935. This was a more radical resection carried out in two stages (see Figure). He advocated a staged operation because of the poor physical status of patients with periampullary tumours coming to surgery: "the victims of these tumors are as a rule deeply jaundiced, have a hemorrhagic diathesis, are depleted, undernourished, asthenic, and have severe liver damage". The first stage consisted of a gastroenterostomy and internal biliary diversion (ligation of the common bile duct and anastomosis of the gall bladder to the stomach). The second stage, undertaken two weeks later, involved excision of the second part of the duodenum together with a wedge of the pancreatic head. The duodenal ends and the pancreatic stump were closed and the pancreatic remnant was not re-implanted. The patient developed a pancreatic leak but eventually recovered. He died from liver metastases 25 months later. All of these pancreatic operations were performed under spinal anaesthesia.

Whipple acknowledged the contribution of others to the concept of excising the duodenum and head of the pancreas in the treatment of periampullary cancer. These included Halsted (1852–1922), who had successfully undertaken local excision of a periampullary carcinoma in 1898 and Kausch (1867–1928), who had reported successful excision of the duodenum and part of the pancreas for ampullary cancer in a two-stage operation in 1912, the patient surviving nine months with no evidence of tumour recurrence at autopsy. He also noted that Lester Dragstedt (1893–1975) had demonstrated the feasibility of total duodenectomy and pancreatic duct ligation in dogs in 1918. It is now believed that pancreaticoduodenectomy was probably first performed in 1898 by the Italian surgeon, Alessandro Codivilla (1861–1912). His patient survived 24 days.

Many variations of the operation followed, including a one-stage pancreaticoduodenectomy by Whipple himself in 1940 for what proved to be a non-functioning islet cell carcinoma. From 1942 onwards, Whipple modified the operation to include partial gastrectomy with gastrojejunostomy, choledochojejunostomy, and re-implantation of the pancreatic duct into a jejunal loop. Whipple performed 37

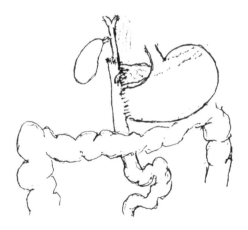

Freehand drawing by Whipple of re-established gastrointestinal continuity following pancreaticoduodenectomy in patients operated on by him after 1942. (From Whipple AO. A reminiscence: pancreaticoduodenectomy. *Rev Surg* 1963;**20**:221–5, Fig.2, p.224. © Elsevier Inc)

pancreaticoduodenectomies during his career, 30 for cancers and seven for chronic pancreatitis. Modifications of the operation led to the development of the modern day 'Whipple' pancreaticoduodenectomy, in which the head and neck of the pancreas, distal stomach, proximal duodenum, gall bladder and common bile duct are resected en bloc; reconstruction is performed with choledochojejunal and pancreatico-jejunal anastomoses. In recent years, a pylorus-preserving technique has been adopted by many surgeons. In specialist units, perioperative mortality from this previously high-risk procedure has fallen below 2%.

Whipple is also remembered for his diagnostic triad associated with insulinoma. 'Whipple's triad' consists of an abnormally low fasting blood sugar, initiation of symptoms by fasting, and relief following the administration of glucose. His name should not be confused with Whipple's disease, an infective disorder of the small intestine causing malabsorption, named after George Whipple (1878–1976), a Nobel prize-winning American physician and pathologist.

Allen Oldfather Whipple (1881–1963)

Whipple was the son of Christian missionaries serving in Persia (now Iran), where he grew up learning to speak English, French, Armenian, Syriac, Turkish and Persian. His father died whilst he was a teenager, leaving him to support himself through college. He attended Princeton University and then Columbia College of Physicians and Surgeons in New York, and gained his MD in 1908. Three years later he was appointed to the faculty at Columbia–Presbyterian Medical Center in New York,

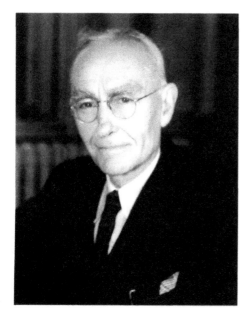

Allen Oldfather Whipple in 1944. (Courtesy of Dr Samir Johna, Department of Surgery, Loma Linda University School of Medicine, California)

where he became Professor of Surgery in 1921 and subsequently Surgeon-in-Chief. He led the department of Surgery for more than 25 years, specialising not only in pancreatic surgery but also in portal hypertension and vascular surgery. Whipple retired in 1946 but remained active in surgical education and research into the history of medicine. On the subject of retirement, he wrote: "Avoid above all else the tragedy of becoming an unoccupied, degenerating vegetable."

Whipple was President of the New York Surgical Society (1934) and Chairman of the American Board of Surgery (1940). He was a trustee of Princeton University and was awarded an honorary Doctorate of Science from Princeton. One of his most treasured honours was the Bigelow Medal awarded by the Boston Surgical Society in 1941. In contrast, a medal he never prized was one that was sent to him from Adolf Hitler for taking care of four German officers who were badly burned when the Hindenburg airship exploded in 1937. After World War II, Whipple also played a key role in the development of hospital care in Iran through his work with the Iran Foundation. In later years, he became an accomplished medical historian and contributed significantly to the understanding of the history of medicine in the Middle East during the Middle Ages.

Whipple's family life was beset by several tragedies, including the death of his 16-year-old son Bill in 1933 in a motor vehicle crash and the sudden loss of his other son from acute liver failure, just eight days before his own death. Whipple died from ischaemic heart disease (personal communication, Dr Samir Johna, Loma Linda University School of Medicine, California) and not from pancreatic cancer, which was reported in one source.

References

Whipple AO, Parsons WB, Mullins CR. Treatment of carcinoma of the ampulla of Vater. *Ann Surg* 1935;**102**:763–79.

Whipple AO. A reminiscence: pancreaticoduodenectomy. *Review of Surgery* 1963;**20**:221–5.

Further reading

Fernández-del Castillo C, Warshaw AL. Surgical pioneers of the pancreas. *Am J Surg* 2007;**194**(Suppl):S2–5.

Johna S. Allen Oldfather Whipple: A distinguished surgeon and historian. *Dig Surg* 2003;**20**:154–62.

Johna S, Schein M. *The Memoirs of Allen Oldfather Whipple. The Man Behind the Whipple Operation.* TFM Publishing Ltd., Shropshire, UK, 2003.

Whipple AO. Philosophy of retirement. *JAMA* 1956;**162**:1043–4.

Whipple AO. The surgical therapy of hyperinsulinism. *Journal de International Chirurgie* 1938;**3**:237–76.

Allen Oldfather Whipple. http://genweb.whipple.org/d0422/I24559.html (Last accessed December 2008).

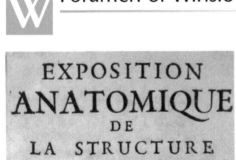

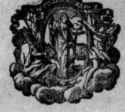

Title page from Winslow JB. *Exposition Anatomique de la Structure du Corps Humain.* Volume 4. Guillaume Desprez et Jean Desessartz, Paris, 1732. (Reproduced with permission of Leeds University Library, UK)

The foramen of Winslow, known as the epiploic foramen, is a short, vertically flat passage connecting the lesser sac with the greater peritoneal cavity. Its boundaries are as follows: anteriorly, the free margin of the lesser omentum containing the bile duct (right) and the hepatic artery proper (left) anterior to the portal vein; superiorly, the caudate process of the liver; posteriorly, the inferior vena cava; and inferiorly, the duodenum and head of pancreas.

Between 1711 and 1743 Winslow published nearly 30 treatises on a variety of subjects. In one of these (1715) he described the foramen between the greater and lesser sacs of the peritoneum. Winslow published his *Exposition Anatomique de la Structure du Corps Humain* in 1732, an authoritative four-volume text on human anatomy that was translated into English, German, Italian and Latin (Winslow 1732). In this, he described "…an opening wide enough to admit the end of the finger". He demonstrated that this foramen communicated with the lesser sac by inserting a pipe into its opening and insufflating air.

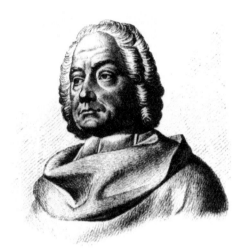

Jacques-Bénigne Winslow.

Jacques-Bénigne Winslow (1669–1760)

Jacob Christian Winslow (later known as Jacques-Bénigne Winslow) was born in Odense in Denmark, the eldest of 13 children of Peder Jakopsen Winslow, Dean of the Protestant Church of Our Lady. Initially Jacob planned to follow family tradition by joining the clergy and in 1687 began studying theology at the University of Copenhagen. However, he soon turned his attentions to anatomy and between 1691 and 1696 Winslow remained in Copenhagen working under the barber-surgeon, Johannes de Buchwald (1658–1738). In 1697 he was awarded a royal scholarship and moved to the Netherlands, where he studied anatomy, clinical medicine, surgery, and obstetrics. Thereafter, he continued his anatomical studies in Paris with the French anatomist, Joseph Guichard Duverney (1648–1730).

Soon after this, at the age of 30 years, Winslow converted to Roman Catholicism, taking his baptismal name Bénigne from Jacques-Bénigne Bousset, Bishop of Meaux. This religious conversion was disapproved of by both the King of Denmark, who terminated Winslow's scholarship, and by Winslow's Lutheran family, who promptly disowned him. He never returned to Denmark.

Duverney made Winslow his assistant in anatomy and surgery at the Jardin du Roi in Paris and in 1705 he was awarded a doctorate of medicine by the University of Paris. Two years later, he was elected to the Royal Academy of Sciences. In addition to his work in anatomy, Winslow maintained a busy medical practice and was appointed Physician at the Hôpital Général, and also at Bicêtre in 1709. In 1743 he became Full Professor of Anatomy at the Jardin du Roi, a post he held until 1758, when he had to retire because of extreme deafness.

211

Winslow remained in Paris for the rest of his life. In 1711, he married Maria Catharina Gilles, with whom he had two children but their son died in early childhood. Winslow is buried in the church of St Benoit in Paris.

Winslow made numerous major contributions to anatomy. He introduced the term 'sympathetic' to describe that part of the autonomic nervous system and he provided a detailed description of the oblique popliteal ligament (of Winslow). He is also remembered for his concern about the then unreliable means of certifying death and the risk of being buried alive. In 1740, he wrote "Death is certain, since it is inevitable, but also uncertain, since its diagnosis is sometimes fallible". He published a detailed compendium of alleged cases of premature burial that helped to promote measures to eliminate this risk.

References

Winslow, JB. *Exposition Anatomique de la Structure du Corps Humain.* Volume 4. Guillaume Desprez et Jean Desessartz, Paris, 1732, pp145–55.

Further reading

Blair DM. Winslow and the sympathetic system. *BMJ* 1932;**2**:1200.

Enersen OD. Jacob Benignus Winslow. www.whonamedit.com (Last accessed July 2005).

Maar V. *L'Autobiographie de Jacques Bénigne Winslow.* Octave Doin & Fils, Paris, 1912.

Winslow JB. *An Anatomical Exposition of the Structure of the Human Body.* (Two volumes in one). Translated from the French original by G. Douglas. Publishers: R Ware and J & P Knapton, London, 1743 (Foramen described in section VIII, p.171).

Winslow JB. The uncertainty of the signs of death, and the danger of precipitate interments and dissections, demonstrated, ... To the whole is added, a curious and entertaining account of the funeral solemnities of many ancient and modern nations, ... A translation by J.J. Bruhier d'Ablaincourt of '*Dissertation sur l'Incertitude des Signes de la Mort*'. M. Cooper, London, 1746.

Wirsüng's duct

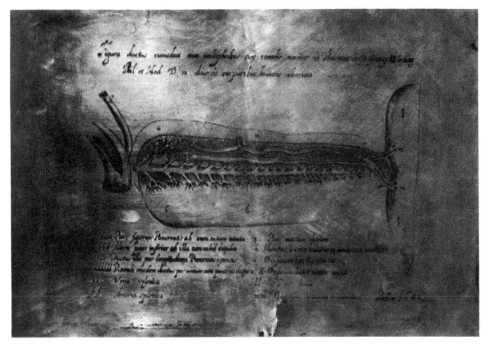

Copper plate engraving of the pancreatic duct produced by Johann Georg Wirsüng at the University of Padua in 1642. The original engraving is now located in the Bo Palace in Padua. (Reproduced with permission of the University of Padua). The inscription reads "Figure of a duct with multiple small branches, recently discovered by Jo.Georg.Wirsüng, doctor of philosophy and medicine, in several human bodies. aaa, upper part of pancreas, not incised, intact; bbb, other, inferior part, considerably retracted from the former; ccc, the duct, extending along the pancreas; dddddd, little branches of this duct, dispersed over the whole pancreas; ee, splenic vein; ff, splenic artery; g, part of the duodenum; h, duct of the gall bladder, entering the duodenum; i, orifice of this duct; k, orifice of the newly discovered duct; ll, part of the spleen; mm, entry of the vessels into the spleen. (Latin translation of copper plate engraving from Howard et al. 1998). Wirsüng made and distributed seven imprints from this copper plate.

In Italy in 1642, the year Galileo died, Wirsüng dissected a pancreatic duct in a 30-year-old man who had been hanged for murder. The dissection was performed privately at San Francesco Hospital and not in the famous anatomy theatre at the University of Padua. Wirsüng realised the significance of his finding and recorded his observations with a single copper plate engraving. He promptly sent copies of the engraving to several famous anatomists in Europe, including Jean Riolan the Younger, his former professor in Paris, enquiring about the possible function of the duct. He did not receive a single reply. More than a year later, and just six weeks before his death, he again wrote to Riolan stating that he had found the duct not only in human adults, newborns and fetuses but also in a variety of animals.

213

Legend has it that there was considerable argument among students and physicians over whether the duct should be named after Wirsüng or a German student, Moritz Hoffman (1622–1698). Hoffman, who later became Professor of Anatomy and Surgery at the University of Altdorf in Germany, had been present at the dissection of the pancreatic duct by Wirsüng in 1642, along with Thomas Bartholin (1616–1680) from Denmark. Five years after Wirsüng's death, Hoffman claimed that he had discovered the duct in 1641 in a turkey rooster and had shared this unpublished finding with Wirsüng.

The discovery of the pancreatic duct by Wirsüng demonstrated that the pancreas was a secretory gland that emptied into the duodenum. Its function until then had been uncertain. Regnier de Graaf (1641–1673) is purported to have been the first to cannulate the pancreatic duct, which he did in dogs.

Johann Georg Wirsüng (1589–1643)

Wirsüng was born in Augsburg in 1589 and studied anatomy at the University of Paris under Professor Jean Riolan the Younger (1577–1657) and in Altdorf. In 1629 he enrolled at the University of Padua in Italy. The University of Padua, founded in 1222, was the leading university for anatomical studies in Europe at that time. Andreas Vesalius (1514–1564) and Gabriele Fallopio (1523–1562) were numbered among its medical luminaries and Galileo (1564–1642) had been Professor of

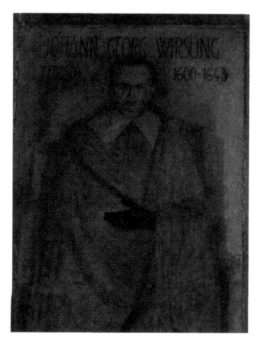

There is no known engraving or painting of Wirsüng. In the Sala dei Quaranta, the old Main Assembly Hall (Aula Magna) of the Bo Palace in Padua there is a symbolic or idealised portrait of Wirsüng painted by Giacomo dal Forno in 1942. (Reproduction of this image strictly licensed by the Università degli Studi di Padova)

Mathematics there. The language of instruction was Latin. Wirsüng graduated from the University of Padua in 1630, with a doctorate in philosophy and medicine and was subsequently appointed Prosector of Anatomy at the University.

On 22 August 1643, at about midnight, Wirsüng was standing in the doorway of his residence talking to fellow tenants when he was shot and killed by a Belgian student, Jacques Cambier. Numerous authors have tried to link this quarrel to the issue of priority concerning the discovery of the pancreatic duct but Giovanni Batista Morgagni (1682–1771), another famous anatomist at the University of Padua, described the incident in detail a century later and concluded that Wirsüng was killed as a result of a private quarrel, the likes of which often arose between young foreign students. Cambier fled from Padua along with his two accomplices the day after the murder.

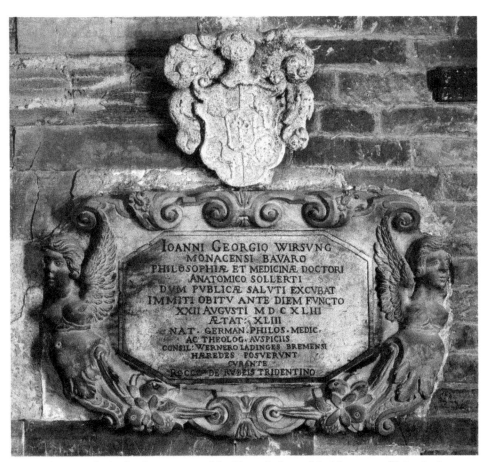

Wirsüng's cenotaph. (By kind permission of the Photo Archive of the Messenger of Saint Anthony. © Deganello Giorgio, Padua, Italy)

Wirsüng was buried in the Chapter Courtyard of St Anthony's Basilica in Padua, where a coat-of-arms marks his cenotaph. A copy of the original marble cenotaph exists in the Palazzo Bo in Padua. Although his cenotaph indicates that he was born in 1600, he almost certainly falsified his age and birthplace (which he gave as Munich) when he enrolled at the University of Padua. This was not uncommon at the time. Europe was in the throes of the Counter-Reformation and Padua and Munich were Catholic cities whereas Augsburg was dominantly Protstant.

References

Howard JM, Hess W, Traverso W. Johann Georg Wirsüng (1589–1643) and the pancreatic duct: the prosector of Padua, Italy. *J Am Coll Surg* 1998;**187**:201–11.

Further reading

Carter M. Assassination of Johann Georg Wirsüng (1589–1643): mysterious medical murder in renaissance Padua. *World J Surg* 1998;**22**:324–6.

Flati G, Andren-Sandberg A. Wirsüng and Santorini: the men behind the ducts. *Pancreatology* 2002;**2**:4–11.

Howard JM, Hess W. *History of the Pancreas. Mysteries of a Hidden Organ.* Springer, Heidelberg, 2002, pp16–30.

McClusky III DA, Skandalakis LJ, Colborn GL, Skandalakis JE. Harbinger or Hermit? Pancreatic anatomy and surgery through the ages – Part 1. *World J Surg* 2002;**26**:1175–85.

Premuda L, Camba A. Per la biografia di Johann Georg Wirsüng e per la storia della scoperta del dotto pancreatico. *Acta Medicae Historiae Patavina* 1974–75;**21**:53–88(Italian).

Schirmer AM. Beitrag zur Geschichte und Anatomie des Pankreas. Inaugural Dissertation behufs Erlangung der Doctorwürde der Hohen Medizinischen. Fäkultät zu Basle vorgelegt Von Alfred Max Schirmer, Praktz. Zahnarzt. L Reinhardt, Universitätsdruckerei, Basle, 1893.

Wood M. Eponyms in biliary tract surgery. *Am J Surg* 1979;**138**:746–54.

Index

Index

219

Index

Index